Heart Healthy Cookbook for Beginners

1800 Days of Simple, Delicious, Low-Sodium, Low Cholesterol & Low-Fat Heart Healthy Recipes for Beginners With a 4-Week Meal Plan for Lowering Blood Pressure and Boosting Heart Health

Alanna Elliott

Table of Contents

INTRODUCTION

Embarking on a path towards better health often begins at the heart of our homes: the kitchen. The foods we choose to prepare and consume play a critical role in the overall function and wellness of our cardiovascular system. A heart-healthy diet is not just a tool for weight management; it's a sustainable approach to living that can improve blood pressure, cholesterol levels, and reduce the risk of heart disease.

This cookbook is dedicated to anyone who wants to embrace a lifestyle that supports heart health through nourishment. The recipes within these pages are crafted with the understanding that food can be both medicine and a source of great joy. We will explore ingredients rich in nutrients that are known to benefit the heart, such as leafy greens, whole grains, and fatty fish, while also learning to reduce the intake of harmful elements like excess sodium and unhealthy fats.

Moreover, this guide is about breaking the myth that healthy eating means sacrificing flavor. On the contrary, it demonstrates how a palette of vibrant fruits, vegetables, whole grains, and lean proteins can come together to create meals that are as delicious as they are beneficial for your heart.

As we navigate the principles of a heart-healthy diet, we'll delve into how to select, prepare, and enjoy foods that contribute to the vitality of your cardiovascular system. This includes understanding labels, balancing macronutrients, and mastering cooking techniques that preserve and enhance nutritional content.

This is not a fad or a temporary fix—it's a commitment to living better, one meal at a time. Whether you are trying to improve your health, maintain it, or simply seeking delicious recipes that are good for your heart, this cookbook is your companion in crafting meals that satisfy your taste buds and support your well-being. Let's bring health to the table with every dish we make.

CHAPTER 1: A COMPREHENSIVE GUIDE TO NOURISHING YOUR CARDIOVASCULAR WELL-BEING

The Importance of a Heart-Healthy Diet

The concept of a heart-healthy diet has gained tremendous traction over the years, and for good reason. It's a response to the growing understanding of how deeply our diet influences cardiac health. The heart is the engine of the human body, pumping blood to every cell and keeping the rhythm of life going. What we eat plays a pivotal role in ensuring this engine runs smoothly and efficiently.

The Direct Impact on Heart Health

At the forefront of a heart-healthy diet is its direct impact on the risk factors for cardiovascular disease, the leading cause of death globally. A diet low in saturated and trans fats, cholesterol, and sodium can help lower blood pressure and cholesterol levels, which are primary contributors to heart disease. Moreover, by integrating a variety of fruits, vegetables, whole grains, and lean proteins into our diet, we can bolster our body's ability to ward off heart-related illnesses.

Weight Management

Obesity and being overweight are significant risk factors for heart disease. A heart-healthy diet typically emphasizes nutrient-dense foods that are lower in calories but high in essential vitamins and minerals. This approach helps in managing weight by promoting fullness with fewer calories, which is crucial in preventing and managing obesity.

Blood Sugar Regulation

The relationship between diet and diabetes is well-documented, with diabetes being a major risk factor for heart disease. A diet that is rich in fiber from whole grains and low in refined sugars helps to slow down the absorption of sugar in your bloodstream, aiding in blood sugar control and insulin sensitivity.

Overall Well-being

Beyond the physical benefits, a heart-healthy diet can also improve mental health and quality of life. Diets rich in omega-3 fatty acids, for example, have been linked to reduced rates of depression, a condition that has its own ties to heart disease. Furthermore, the act of preparing and consuming nutritious foods can be a source of pleasure and can promote a sense of well-being.

Inflammation Reduction

Chronic inflammation is a known trigger for heart disease. Many heart-healthy foods are also anti-inflammatory, like leafy greens, nuts, and fatty fish rich in omega-3 fatty acids. By reducing inflammation, a heart-healthy diet not only helps prevent damage to blood vessels but also supports overall immune function and health.

Longevity and Quality of Life

Adopting a heart-healthy diet isn't just about adding years to life; it's about adding life to years. By reducing the risk of heart disease and its associated conditions, such as stroke, we can improve our chances of living a longer, more active life free from the limitations these diseases can cause.

Empowerment Through Education

Understanding the benefits of a heart-healthy diet empowers individuals to make informed choices about their nutrition. This book aims not just to instruct but also to enlighten, offering the knowledge necessary to decode nutrition labels, understand the body's needs, and make dietary decisions that prioritize heart health.

In conclusion, a heart-healthy diet is more than a collection of food choices. It's a powerful intervention that can transform our health prospects. It's an evidence-based, delicious, and life-enriching path to ensuring that the heart continues to do its vital work with vigor and resilience. With every meal, we have the opportunity to offer our hearts the care and support they deserve.

Understanding Heart Health: Cholesterol, Blood Pressure, and Beyond

At the core of heart health are several critical factors that many of us have heard about: cholesterol, blood pressure, and other less-discussed elements like inflammation and triglycerides. Each of these plays a significant role in the overall health of our cardiovascular system and can be profoundly influenced by our diet and lifestyle choices.

Cholesterol is often at the center of the heart health conversation. It's a waxy, fat-like substance found in all cells of the body. While it's essential for making hormones, vitamin D, and substances that help you digest foods, too much cholesterol can be harmful. It's important to understand the difference between LDL (low-density lipoprotein) cholesterol, often referred to as 'bad' cholesterol, which can build up and clog your arteries, and HDL (high-density lipoprotein) cholesterol, often dubbed the 'good' cholesterol, which helps remove other forms of cholesterol from your bloodstream.

Blood pressure is the force exerted by circulating blood on the walls of blood vessels. Maintaining normal blood pressure is crucial as high blood pressure, or hypertension, forces the heart to work harder than normal, leading to potential damage over time. Hypertension often has no warning signs or symptoms, and many people do not know they have it, which is why it's often called the "silent killer."

Inflammation in the body is a natural response to injury or infection, but when inflammation is chronic, it can lead to the development of plaque in the arteries, known as atherosclerosis. This is a condition where the arteries narrow and harden, which can eventually lead to heart attacks and strokes.

Triglycerides are another type of fat found in the blood. When you eat, your body converts any calories it doesn't need to use right away into triglycerides, which are stored in your fat cells. High levels of triglycerides can contribute to the hardening or thickening of the arterial walls, increasing the risk of stroke, heart attack, and heart disease.

Beyond these familiar terms, heart health is also influenced by a host of other factors, such as blood sugar levels, the balance of electrolytes like potassium and sodium, and even the health of your gut microbiome. Each of these elements can contribute to your cardiovascular health in complex ways.

Understanding these facets of heart health highlights why a well-rounded, nutritious diet is so vital. Foods high in soluble fiber can help lower LDL cholesterol, while those rich in omega-3 fatty acids can reduce inflammation and triglyceride levels. Foods low in sodium and rich in potassium can help manage blood pressure. In essence, a heart-healthy diet is not just about subtracting the bad, but also about adding the good—nutrients that support the body's natural processes and promote overall health.

As we navigate through the intricacies of diet and its impact on these elements, it becomes clear that a proactive approach to eating can help us maintain not just a healthy heart, but a healthy body overall.

Key Components of Heart-Healthy Foods

The foundation of a heart-healthy diet is built upon foods that work together to bolster cardiovascular function, support blood vessel health, and reduce the risk of heart disease. These components, ranging from macro to micronutrients, serve as the building blocks for meals that are not just nourishing but also protective of one of our most vital organs.

Fiber

Fiber is a star in heart-healthy eating. Soluble fiber, found in foods like oats, flaxseeds, beans, lentils, and certain fruits, helps to lower LDL (bad) cholesterol by binding to it in the digestive system and removing it from the body. Insoluble fiber, present in whole grains, nuts, and vegetables, aids in digestion and helps to keep you full, which can assist in weight management.

Whole Grains

Whole grains are integral to a heart-healthy diet. Unlike their refined counterparts, whole grains are rich in nutrients and have all parts of the grain intact, which means they provide more fiber, B vitamins, and minerals like iron, selenium, and magnesium. Studies have shown that consuming whole grains can lead to a lower risk of heart disease.

Healthy Fats

Fats are essential, but the type of fat is what's important. Monounsaturated and polyunsaturated fats — found in olive oil, avocados, nuts, and fatty fish — can help reduce the risk of heart disease when used in place of saturated and trans fats. Omega-3 fatty acids, a type of polyunsaturated fat, are particularly beneficial and have been linked to a decreased risk of arrhythmias (abnormal heartbeats) and atherosclerosis (plaque build-up in the arteries). They also help lower triglyceride levels.

Fruits and Vegetables

Fruits and vegetables are high in vitamins, minerals, and antioxidants — and they're low in calories. Rich in dietary fiber, they help to lower blood pressure and LDL cholesterol. They are also abundant in potassium, which is key in controlling blood pressure.

Lean Proteins

A heart-healthy diet includes lean proteins such as poultry, fish, beans, and legumes. These proteins have less saturated fat than red meat. Fish, like salmon and mackerel, are high in omega-3 fatty acids, which have heart-protective benefits.

Low-Fat Dairy

Low-fat dairy products provide calcium and protein, but it's important to choose versions that are low in saturated fat. These can help to maintain bone health without negatively impacting blood cholesterol levels.

Sodium

Keeping sodium intake low is crucial for heart health. Excessive sodium can lead to high blood pressure, a risk factor for cardiovascular disease. Heart-healthy eating involves choosing fresh, unprocessed foods that are naturally low in sodium and using herbs and spices for flavoring instead of salt.

Antioxidants

Antioxidants found in a variety of foods, particularly in colorful fruits and vegetables, can protect your heart by reducing oxidative stress and inflammation. These include vitamins C and E, selenium, and carotenoids, such as beta-carotene.

Plant Sterols and Stanols

These substances, which are found naturally in plants, help block the absorption of cholesterol in the body. They can be found in certain fortified foods and dietary supplements, and consuming them as part of a balanced diet can help to lower LDL cholesterol.

Incorporating these components into a daily eating plan doesn't have to be difficult. It's about making simple, consistent choices—opting for whole grains over refined ones, snacking on a piece of fruit instead of processed foods, choosing a handful of nuts over chips, and selecting lean meats and fish instead of high-fat cuts. By focusing on these key elements, a heart-healthy diet becomes not just a means to support cardiovascular health, but a pleasurable way of eating that can be maintained for life.

How to Read Nutritional Labels for Heart Health

Understanding nutritional labels is crucial for maintaining a heart-healthy diet. These labels are your guide to making choices that benefit your heart and overall health. The first thing to look at is the serving size, which can be very different from the portion you might typically eat. All the information on the label is based on this amount, so if you eat double the serving size, you're also getting double the calories, fat, sodium, and other components listed.

Calories are a measure of energy, and balancing calories consumed with calories burned is fundamental to maintaining a healthy weight. However, the quality of those calories matters immensely for heart health. Lower-calorie doesn't always mean healthier, especially if those calories come from sugar or trans fats rather than from whole grains and lean proteins.

The fats section is divided into saturated, unsaturated, and trans fats. Saturated and trans fats are the ones to limit for heart health, as they can raise your bad cholesterol levels. Look for foods that have higher amounts of monounsaturated and polyunsaturated fats, which can actually be beneficial for your cholesterol levels.

Cholesterol and sodium are next on the label. Keeping these numbers low is key, as too much cholesterol can lead to plaque buildup in your arteries, and too much sodium can contribute to high blood pressure. Remember that the daily recommended maximum for sodium is less than 2,300 milligrams, though lower is better, especially for those with hypertension.

1500 sodium

Fiber is a nutrient that many people don't get enough of. High-fiber foods are important for heart health because fiber helps to lower cholesterol and can make you feel full, which helps with weight management. Look for foods with a high dietary fiber content per serving.

Sugars, now often listed as "total sugars" and "added sugars," can be tricky. Natural sugars occur in many nutritious foods like fruits and dairy, but added sugars are the ones to watch out for. Consuming too much added sugar can lead to weight gain and increased triglyceride levels, which are risk factors for heart disease.

Proteins are essential for various bodily functions, and getting enough protein can help maintain muscle mass and aid in weight management. However, the source of protein is important; lean proteins are preferred for heart health.

The vitamins and minerals section will often list vitamin D, calcium, iron, and potassium. Potassium can help counteract the effects of sodium and help lower blood pressure, so foods high in potassium are good for heart health. *Potatoes- bananas.*

Lastly, ingredient lists tell you what's in the food, starting with the largest component first. Look for whole food ingredients and be cautious of long lists with unrecognizable items, which can often mean unnecessary additives.

Learning to read and understand food labels means you can make informed decisions about what you eat, which will help you control the factors that contribute to heart health such as cholesterol, blood pressure, and weight.

Tips for Heart-Healthy Cooking and Meal Planning

Adopting a heart-healthy approach to cooking and meal planning requires a shift in perspective and a willingness to embrace new methods and ingredients. These tips are designed to help make this transition seamless and enjoyable, ensuring that meals not only nourish the heart but also delight the palate.

Start with Whole Foods
Base your meals on whole, unprocessed ingredients. Vegetables, fruits, whole grains, nuts, and legumes should fill most of your plate. These foods are naturally low in sodium, high in fiber, and packed with nutrients that support heart health.

Cook with Healthy Fats
Use oils that are rich in monounsaturated and polyunsaturated fats, like olive oil, canola oil, or avocado oil, instead of butter or lard. When cooking at high temperatures, use oils with a high smoke point to prevent harmful compounds from forming.

Increase Fiber Intake
Incorporate more high-fiber foods into your meals. Whole grains like quinoa, brown rice, and

whole-wheat pasta, legumes such as beans and lentils, and a variety of vegetables and fruits can all contribute to the necessary fiber your body needs to manage cholesterol and improve digestive health.

Select Lean Proteins

Choose lean meats such as poultry and fish. Remove skin and visible fat from meat to reduce saturated fat intake. Including plant-based proteins like beans, lentils, and tofu can also provide high-quality protein with less saturated fat and more fiber.

Incorporate Omega-3s

Regularly eat fish high in omega-3 fatty acids, such as salmon, trout, and herring. Plant sources of omega-3s include flaxseeds, chia seeds, and walnuts. These fats are vital for heart health, particularly in managing inflammation and maintaining a healthy heart rhythm.

Cut Down on Salt

Reduce the amount of salt used in cooking. Experiment with herbs, spices, citrus, and vinegar to add flavor without the need for extra sodium. Be mindful of the salt content in prepackaged spice blends and sauces, opting for fresh or dried herbs as alternatives.

Be Smart About Dairy

Choose low-fat or fat-free dairy products to reduce the intake of saturated fats while maintaining a good source of calcium and protein. Greek yogurt, for instance, can be a versatile ingredient for both sweet and savory dishes.

Control Portion Sizes

Keep an eye on portion sizes to avoid overeating, which can lead to weight gain and negatively affect heart health. Using smaller plates can help, and be sure to fill half your plate with vegetables, a quarter with lean protein, and the remaining quarter with whole grains.

Plan Your Meals

Planning meals in advance can help you make healthier choices and avoid last-minute decisions that might lead to less healthy options. It also makes grocery shopping more efficient and can reduce food waste.

Practice Healthy Cooking Methods

Instead of frying, choose to grill, broil, roast, steam, or bake your food. These cooking methods do not require large amounts of added fat and can help retain the nutrients in your food.

Manage Your Portions and Leftovers

Learn to listen to your hunger cues and eat until you're satisfied, not stuffed. Embrace leftovers, which can save time and energy while also helping you stick to your heart-healthy eating plan.

By incorporating these strategies into your daily routine, cooking and eating for heart health can become a natural part of your lifestyle. Over time, these habits can have a profound impact on your cardiovascular well-being, as well as on your overall health and enjoyment of food.

CHAPTER 2: BREAKFAST

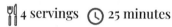

Oatmeal with Blueberries and Chia Seeds

🍴 4 servings 🕐 25 minutes

INGREDIENTS
- 2 cups rolled oats
- 4 cups water (or a mixture of water and your choice of milk for creaminess)
- 1 cup fresh blueberries
- 2 tablespoons chia seeds
- 1 teaspoon vanilla extract
- 2 tablespoons honey or pure maple syrup (optional)
- 1/4 teaspoon cinnamon (optional)
- A pinch of salt

DIRECTIONS
1. In a medium saucepan, bring the 4 cups of water (or water-milk mixture) to a boil. Add a pinch of salt.
2. Stir in the rolled oats and simmer on low heat, stirring occasionally, for about 10-15 minutes or until the oats have absorbed the liquid and reached your desired consistency.
3. Remove from heat and stir in the vanilla extract, cinnamon (if using), and honey or maple syrup (if using).
4. Let the oatmeal sit for a couple of minutes to cool slightly; it will thicken upon standing.
5. Stir in the chia seeds and allow them to sit for a few minutes to swell and soften.
6. Serve the oatmeal in bowls topped with fresh blueberries.

Nutritional Information per serving: Calories: 210 | Total Fat: 4.5g | Saturated Fat: 0.5g | Trans Fat: 0g | Polyunsaturated Fat: 3g | Monounsaturated Fat: 1g | Cholesterol: 0mg | Sodium: 60mg | Carbohydrates: 37g | Fiber: 7g | Sugars: 7g | Protein: 6g

Avocado Toast on Whole Grain Bread

🍴 2 servings 🕐 5 minutes

INGREDIENTS
- 1 ripe avocado
- 2 slices of whole grain bread
- 1 small tomato, sliced
- 1/2 lemon, juiced
- Salt and pepper to taste
- Red pepper flakes (optional)
- 1 teaspoon chia seeds (optional)

DIRECTIONS
1. Toast the whole grain bread slices to your preferred level of crispiness.
2. Cut the avocado in half, remove the pit, and scoop the flesh into a bowl.
3. Mash the avocado with a fork until it reaches your desired consistency.
4. Mix in the lemon juice, and season with salt and pepper. Add red pepper flakes if you like a bit of heat.
5. Spread the mashed avocado evenly over the toasted bread slices.
6. Top each slice with tomato slices and sprinkle with chia seeds for an extra nutrient boost.
7. Serve immediately and enjoy!

Nutritional Information per serving: Calories: 250 | Total Fat: 15g | Saturated Fat: 2g | Trans Fat: 0g | Polyunsaturated Fat: 2g | Monounsaturated Fat: 10g | Cholesterol: 0mg | Sodium: 200mg | Carbohydrates: 26g | Fiber: 9g | Sugars: 4g | Protein: 6g

Greek Yogurt Parfait with Mixed Berries and Almonds

🍴 4 servings 🕐 10 minutes

INGREDIENTS
- 2 cups plain Greek yogurt (low-fat or fat-free)
- 1 cup mixed berries (such as strawberries, blueberries, raspberries)
- 1/2 cup almonds, sliced or chopped
- 4 teaspoons honey or pure maple syrup
- 1/2 teaspoon vanilla extract (optional)
- A sprinkle of ground cinnamon (optional)

DIRECTIONS
1. If using, mix the vanilla extract into the Greek yogurt in a bowl.
2. In serving glasses or bowls, layer the Greek yogurt and mixed berries.
3. Drizzle each layer with a teaspoon of honey or maple syrup.
4. Top each parfait with sliced or chopped almonds.
5. Optionally, sprinkle a small amount of ground cinnamon on top for added flavor.
6. Serve immediately or refrigerate until ready to serve.

Nutritional Information per serving: Calories: 180 | Total Fat: 6g | Saturated Fat: 0.5g | Trans Fat: 0g | Polyunsaturated Fat: 1.5g | Monounsaturated Fat: 3.5g | Cholesterol: 5mg | Sodium: 45mg | Carbohydrates: 18g | Fiber: 3g | Sugars: 12g | Protein: 15g

Quinoa Breakfast Bowl with Nuts and Apples

🍴 4 servings   🕐 25 minutes

INGREDIENTS

- 1 cup quinoa, rinsed
- 2 cups water
- 1 large apple, cored and chopped
- 1/2 cup walnuts, chopped (or nuts of your choice)
- 1/4 cup raisins or dried cranberries
- 1/2 teaspoon ground cinnamon
- 1/4 teaspoon ground nutmeg
- 2 tablespoons honey or maple syrup
- Optional toppings: a dollop of Greek yogurt, a sprinkle of chia seeds, or a drizzle of almond butter

DIRECTIONS

1. In a medium saucepan, bring 2 cups of water to a boil. Add the rinsed quinoa and a pinch of salt, then reduce heat to low, cover, and simmer for about 15-20 minutes, or until all water is absorbed and the quinoa is fluffy.
2. While the quinoa is cooking, chop the apple and prepare the nuts and other toppings.
3. When the quinoa is done, remove from heat. Stir in the chopped apple, nuts, raisins (or dried cranberries), cinnamon, and nutmeg.
4. Sweeten the mixture with honey or maple syrup, adjusting to your taste.
5. Divide the quinoa mixture into bowls. If desired, top each serving with a dollop of Greek yogurt, a sprinkle of chia seeds, or a drizzle of almond butter.
6. Serve warm, and enjoy!

Nutritional Information per serving: Calories:300 | Total Fat: 9g | Saturated Fat: 1g | Trans Fat: 0g | Polyunsaturated Fat: 5g | Monounsaturated Fat: 2g | Cholesterol: 0mg | Sodium: 10mg | Carbohydrates: 49g | Fiber: 6g | Sugars: 15g | Protein: 8g

Spinach and Mushroom Egg White Omelet

🍴 2 servings   🕐 18 minutes

INGREDIENTS

- 4 large egg whites
- 1 cup fresh spinach, chopped
- 1/2 cup mushrooms, sliced
- 1 small onion, finely chopped
- 2 cloves garlic, minced
- 1/4 cup low-fat feta cheese, crumbled
- 1 teaspoon olive oil
- Salt and pepper to taste
- Fresh herbs (like parsley or chives) for garnish (optional)

DIRECTIONS

1. In a non-stick skillet, heat the olive oil over medium heat. Add the chopped onion and garlic, sautéing until the onion is translucent.
2. Add the sliced mushrooms to the skillet and cook until they are soft and browned.
3. Stir in the chopped spinach and cook until it wilts. Season the mixture with salt and pepper. Transfer the vegetables to a plate and set aside.
4. In a bowl, whisk the egg whites until frothy. Season with a pinch of salt and pepper.
5. In the same skillet, pour in the egg whites. Cook over medium heat until the eggs begin to set around the edges.
6. Gently spread the sautéed vegetables and crumbled feta cheese over one half of the egg whites.
7. Using a spatula, carefully fold the other half of the omelet over the filling. Let it cook for another minute.
8. Slide the omelet onto a plate, garnish with fresh herbs if desired, and serve hot.

Nutritional Information per serving: Calories: 110 | Total Fat: 4g | Saturated Fat: 1g | Trans Fat: 0g | Polyunsaturated Fat: 0.5g | Monounsaturated Fat: 2g | Cholesterol: 5mg | Sodium: 320mg | Carbohydrates: 5g | Fiber: 1g | Sugars: 2g | Protein: 13g

Banana Walnut Overnight Oats

🍴 4 servings   🕐 5 minutes

INGREDIENTS

- 2 cups rolled oats
- 2 ripe bananas, mashed
- 2 tablespoons chia seeds
- 1/2 cup walnuts, chopped
- 2 cups unsweetened almond milk (or milk of choice)
- 1 teaspoon vanilla extract
- 1/2 teaspoon ground cinnamon
- 2 tablespoons honey or maple syrup (optional)

DIRECTIONS

1. In a large bowl, combine the rolled oats, mashed bananas, chia seeds, and chopped walnuts.

2. Add the almond milk, vanilla extract, and ground cinnamon. Stir well to ensure all ingredients are thoroughly mixed.
3. If you prefer a bit of added sweetness, stir in honey or maple syrup.
4. Divide the mixture evenly into jars or airtight containers. Seal and place in the refrigerator overnight (or for at least 6 hours).
5. In the morning, give the oats a good stir. If the mixture is too thick, add a little more milk to reach your desired consistency.
6. Serve cold or heat up in the microwave if preferred. Enjoy!

Nutritional Information per serving: Calories: 355 | Total Fat: 14g | Saturated Fat: 1.5g | Trans Fat: 0g | Polyunsaturated Fat: 7g | Monounsaturated Fat: 3g | Cholesterol: 0mg | Sodium: 60mg | Carbohydrates: 52g | Fiber: 9g | Sugars: 11g | Protein: 11g.

Smoked Salmon and Avocado Whole Wheat Bagel

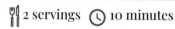 2 servings 🕐 10 minutes

INGREDIENTS

- 2 whole wheat bags, halved
- 4 ounces smoked salmon
- 1 ripe avocado
- 1 tablespoon capers
- 1/2 small red onion, thinly sliced
- 2 tablespoons low-fat cream cheese (or Greek yogurt)
- Fresh dill for garnish
- Freshly ground black pepper
- Lemon wedges for serving

DIRECTIONS

1. Toast the whole wheat bagel halves until they are lightly browned and crispy.
2. Peel and slice the avocado. Set aside.
3. Spread each bagel half with a tablespoon of low-fat cream cheese or Greek yogurt.
4. Place a few slices of smoked salmon on each bagel half.
5. Add sliced avocado on top of the salmon.
6. Sprinkle capers and red onion slices over the avocado.
7. Garnish with fresh dill and a twist of freshly ground black pepper.
8. Serve each bagel with a wedge of lemon on the side.

Nutritional Information per serving: Calories: Approximately 400 | Total Fat: 19g | Saturated Fat: 3g | Trans Fat: 0g | Polyunsaturated Fat: 3g | Monounsaturated Fat: 9g | Cholesterol: 20mg | Sodium: 600mg | Carbohydrates: 38g | Fiber: 7g | Sugars: 5g | Protein: 24g.

Almond Butter and Banana Smoothie

🍴 2 servings 🕐 5 minutes

INGREDIENTS

- 2 ripe bananas
- 2 tablespoons almond butter
- 1 cup unsweetened almond milk
- 1/2 cup Greek yogurt (low-fat or fat-free)
- 1 tablespoon flaxseeds or chia seeds
- 1/2 teaspoon vanilla extract
- A pinch of cinnamon
- Ice cubes (optional)

DIRECTIONS

1. Peel the bananas and place them in a blender.
2. Add the almond butter, almond milk, Greek yogurt, flaxseeds or chia seeds, vanilla extract, and cinnamon.
3. Add a handful of ice cubes if you prefer a colder, thicker smoothie.
4. Blend on high until smooth and creamy.
5. Taste and adjust the sweetness or thickness, if necessary, by adding a bit more almond milk or a sweetener of your choice.
6. Pour into glasses and serve immediately.

Nutritional Information per serving: Calories: Approximately 280 | Total Fat: 14g | Saturated Fat: 1.5g | Trans Fat: 0g | Polyunsaturated Fat: 3g | Monounsaturated Fat: 8g | Cholesterol: 5mg | Sodium: 100mg | Carbohydrates: 30g | Fiber: 5g | Sugars: 16g | Protein: 10g

Kale and Red Pepper Mini Frittatas

🍴 6 servings 🕐 35 minutes

INGREDIENTS

- 6 large egg whites
- 2 whole eggs
- 1 cup kale, chopped and stems removed
- 1 red bell pepper, diced
- 1/2 onion, finely chopped
- 1/4 cup low-fat milk
- 1/4 cup low-fat feta cheese, crumbled
- Salt and pepper to taste
- Non-stick cooking spray or a little olive oil

DIRECTIONS

1. Preheat the oven to 350°F (175°C). Spray a muffin tin with non-stick cooking spray or lightly grease with olive oil.
2. In a skillet, sauté the onions and red bell pepper until softened. Add the kale and cook until it's

wilted. Season with salt and pepper.

3. In a large bowl, whisk together the egg whites, whole eggs, and milk. Season with a pinch of salt and pepper.
4. Add the sautéed vegetables to the egg mixture, then stir in the crumbled feta cheese.
5. Pour the mixture into the prepared muffin tin, filling each cup about 3/4 full.
6. Bake for 20 minutes, or until the frittatas are set and slightly golden on top.
7. Let them cool for a few minutes before removing from the tin. Serve warm.

Nutritional Information per serving: Calories: 90 | Total Fat: 3g | Saturated Fat: 1g | Trans Fat: 0g | Polyunsaturated Fat: 1g | Monounsaturated Fat: 1g | Cholesterol: 65mg | Sodium: 200mg | Carbohydrates: 4g | Fiber: 1g | Sugars: 2g | Protein: 10g

Steel-Cut Oats with Pomegranate Seeds

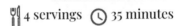 4 servings 🕐 35 minutes

INGREDIENTS
- 1 cup steel-cut oats
- 4 cups water
- 1/2 teaspoon cinnamon
- 1/4 teaspoon nutmeg
- 1 cup pomegranate seeds
- 1/4 cup chopped walnuts or almonds
- Honey or maple syrup (optional, for sweetening)

DIRECTIONS
1. Bring the water to a boil in a large saucepan. Add the steel-cut oats and a pinch of salt, then reduce the heat to low.
2. Simmer the oats, uncovered, for about 25-30 minutes, stirring occasionally, until they reach your desired consistency.
3. Stir in the cinnamon and nutmeg.
4. Serve the oats in bowls, topped with pomegranate seeds and chopped nuts.
5. If desired, drizzle with a little honey or maple syrup for added sweetness.

Nutritional Information per serving: Calories: 220 | Total Fat: 6g | Saturated Fat: 0.5g | Trans Fat: 0g | Polyunsaturated Fat: 2.5g | Monounsaturated Fat: 2g | Cholesterol: 0mg | Sodium: 10mg | Carbohydrates: 36g | Fiber: 6g | Sugars: 8g | Protein: 7g

Chia Seed Pudding with Kiwi and Coconut

🍴 4 servings 🕐 15 minutes

INGREDIENTS
- 1/4 cup chia seeds
- 1 cup unsweetened almond milk
- 1 tablespoon honey or maple syrup (optional)
- 1 teaspoon vanilla extract
- 2 kiwis, peeled and sliced
- 1/4 cup shredded unsweetened coconut

DIRECTIONS
1. In a bowl, mix together the chia seeds, almond milk, honey or maple syrup (if using), and vanilla extract.
2. Stir well and let the mixture sit for 5 minutes. Stir again to prevent clumping.
3. Cover the bowl and refrigerate for at least 2 hours or overnight until it achieves a pudding-like consistency.
4. To serve, layer the chia pudding in glasses with slices of kiwi and top with shredded coconut.

Nutritional Information per serving: Calories: 150 | Total Fat: 7g | Saturated Fat: 3g | Trans Fat: 0g | Polyunsaturated Fat: 2g | Monounsaturated Fat: 1g | Cholesterol: 0mg | Sodium: 45mg | Carbohydrates: 20g | Fiber: 6g | Sugars: 10g | Protein: 4g

Whole Grain Pancakes with Fresh Fruit Compote

🍴 4 servings 🕐 40 minutes

INGREDIENTS
- 1 cup whole grain pancake mix
- 3/4 cup low-fat milk
- 1 egg
- 1 tablespoon canola oil
- 2 cups mixed fresh fruit (berries, sliced peaches, etc.)
- 2 tablespoons water
- 1 tablespoon honey or maple syrup

DIRECTIONS
1. Prepare the pancake batter according to package instructions using the whole grain mix, milk, egg, and oil. Let the batter rest for a few minutes.
2. Heat a non-stick skillet over medium heat and cook pancakes until golden brown on both sides.
3. For the compote, combine the mixed fruit, water, and honey or maple syrup in a saucepan. Simmer over low heat until the fruit is soft and the sauce has thickened.
4. Serve the pancakes topped with the warm fruit compote.

Nutritional Information per serving: Calories: 250 | Total Fat: 6g | Saturated Fat: 1g | Trans Fat: 0g | Polyunsaturated Fat: 2g | Monounsaturated Fat: 2g | Cholesterol: 55mg | Sodium: 150mg | Carbohydrates: 42g | Fiber: 5g | Sugars: 16g | Protein: 8g

Cottage Cheese with Pineapple and Flaxseeds

🍴 4 servings 🕐 5 minutes

INGREDIENTS
- 2 cups low-fat cottage cheese
- 1 cup chopped fresh pineapple
- 2 tablespoons ground flaxseeds

DIRECTIONS
1. Divide the cottage cheese among four bowls.
2. Top each bowl with chopped pineapple and sprinkle with ground flaxseeds.

Nutritional Information per serving: Calories: 180 | Total Fat: 4g | Saturated Fat: 1g | Trans Fat: 0g | Polyunsaturated Fat: 2g | Monounsaturated Fat: 1g | Cholesterol: 10mg | Sodium: 400mg | Carbohydrates: 16g | Fiber: 2g | Sugars: 12g | Protein: 20g

Baked Sweet Potato Hash with Peppers and Onions

🍴 4 servings 🕐 40 minutes

INGREDIENTS
- 2 medium sweet potatoes, peeled and diced
- 1 red bell pepper, diced
- 1 green bell pepper, diced
- 1 onion, diced
- 2 tablespoons olive oil
- Salt and pepper to taste
- 1/2 teaspoon smoked paprika (optional)

DIRECTIONS
1. Preheat the oven to 400°F (200°C). Line a baking sheet with parchment paper.
2. In a large bowl, toss together the diced sweet potatoes, bell peppers, onion, olive oil, salt, pepper, and smoked paprika.
3. Spread the mixture in a single layer on the prepared baking sheet.
4. Bake for 25 minutes, stirring halfway through, until the vegetables are tender and lightly browned.

Nutritional Information per serving: Calories: 180 | Total Fat: 7g | Saturated Fat: 1g | Trans Fat: 0g | Polyunsaturated Fat: 1g | Monounsaturated Fat: 5g | Cholesterol: 0mg | Sodium: 100mg | Carbohydrates: 27g | Fiber: 4g | Sugars: 9g | Protein: 2g

Raspberry Almond Muffins (Made with Oat Flour)

🍴 12 servings 🕐 35 minutes

INGREDIENTS
- 2 cups oat flour
- 1/2 cup almond flour
- 1/2 cup honey or maple syrup
- 1 teaspoon baking powder
- 1/2 teaspoon baking soda
- 1/4 teaspoon salt
- 2 eggs
- 3/4 cup unsweetened almond milk
- 1/4 cup coconut oil, melted
- 1 teaspoon vanilla extract
- 1 cup fresh raspberries
- 1/4 cup sliced almonds

DIRECTIONS
1. Preheat the oven to 350°F (175°C). Line a muffin tin with paper liners.
2. In a large bowl, whisk together oat flour, almond flour, baking powder, baking soda, and salt.
3. In another bowl, beat the eggs with honey, almond milk, melted coconut oil, and vanilla extract.
4. Add the wet ingredients to the dry ingredients and stir until just combined.
5. Gently fold in the raspberries.
6. Divide the batter among the muffin cups and sprinkle the tops with sliced almonds.
7. Bake for 20 minutes or until a toothpick inserted into the center comes out clean.
8. Let the muffins cool before serving.

Nutritional Information per serving: Calories: 220 | Total Fat: 10g | Saturated Fat: 4g | Trans Fat: 0g | Polyunsaturated Fat: 2g | Monounsaturated Fat: 3g | Cholesterol: 31mg | Sodium: 150mg | Carbohydrates: 28g | Fiber: 3g | Sugars: 12g | Protein: 5g.

Turkey and Spinach Breakfast Burritos (Using Whole Wheat Tortillas)

🍴 4 servings 🕐 20 minutes

INGREDIENTS
- 4 whole wheat tortillas
- 8 ounces lean ground turkey
- 2 cups fresh spinach, chopped
- 4 eggs, beaten
- 1/2 cup shredded low-fat cheddar cheese
- 1/4 cup salsa
- Salt and pepper to taste
- Non-stick cooking spray or a small amount of olive oil

DIRECTIONS

1. Heat a non-stick skillet over medium heat. Spray with cooking spray or add a small amount of olive oil.
2. Cook the ground turkey in the skillet until it's no longer pink, breaking it up as it cooks. Season with salt and pepper.
3. Add the chopped spinach to the skillet and cook until it wilts.
4. Pour the beaten eggs over the turkey and spinach mixture. Let the eggs cook for a few seconds and then gently scramble them with the turkey and spinach until fully cooked.
5. Warm the whole wheat tortillas in the microwave for about 20-30 seconds or in a dry skillet over low heat.
6. Divide the turkey, spinach, and egg mixture evenly among the tortillas. Sprinkle each with shredded cheese.
7. Add a tablespoon of salsa to each burrito.
8. Roll up the tortillas, folding in the sides first, and then rolling them up from the bottom to enclose the filling.
9. Serve immediately or wrap in foil to keep warm.

Nutritional Information per serving: Calories: 330 | Total Fat: 15g | Saturated Fat: 5g | Trans Fat: 0g | Polyunsaturated Fat: 3g | Monounsaturated Fat: 5g | Cholesterol: 215mg | Sodium: 640mg | Carbohydrates: 23g | Fiber: 3g | Sugars: 3g | Protein: 27g

Poached Eggs over Sautéed Greens and Whole Grain Toast

🍴 2 servings 🕐 15 minutes

INGREDIENTS

- 2 large eggs
- 2 cups mixed greens (kale, spinach, chard)
- 2 slices whole grain bread
- 1 tablespoon olive oil
- Salt and pepper to taste
- Optional: vinegar for poaching eggs

DIRECTIONS

1. Lightly toast the whole grain bread.
2. Heat olive oil in a pan and sauté the mixed greens until wilted. Season with salt and pepper.
3. To poach the eggs, bring a pot of water to a simmer and add a splash of vinegar. Gently drop the eggs into the water and poach for about 3-4 minutes.
4. Place sautéed greens on toast, top each with a poached egg. Season with salt and pepper to taste.

Nutritional Information per serving: Calories: 250 | Total Fat: 12g | Saturated Fat: 3g | Trans Fat: 0g |

Polyunsaturated Fat: 2g | Monounsaturated Fat: 6g | Cholesterol: 186mg | Sodium: 370mg | Carbohydrates: 23g | Fiber: 4g | Sugars: 3g | Protein: 13g

Berry and Spinach Smoothie with Soy Milk

🍴 2 servings 🕐 5 minutes

INGREDIENTS

- 1 cup fresh spinach
- 1 cup mixed berries (blueberries, strawberries, raspberries)
- 1 banana
- 1 1/2 cups soy milk
- 1 tablespoon honey or maple syrup (optional)

DIRECTIONS

1. Blend spinach, berries, banana, and soy milk until smooth.
2. Add honey or maple syrup for sweetness if desired.

Nutritional Information per serving: Calories: 180 | Total Fat: 3g | Saturated Fat: 0.5g | Trans Fat: 0g | Polyunsaturated Fat: 1.5g | Monounsaturated Fat: 0.5g | Cholesterol: 0mg | Sodium: 95mg | Carbohydrates: 33g | Fiber: 5g | Sugars: 20g | Protein: 7g

Pear and Walnut Baked Oatmeal

🍴 6 servings 🕐 45 minutes

INGREDIENTS

- 2 cups rolled oats
- 1/4 cup walnuts, chopped
- 2 ripe pears, diced
- 1/4 cup honey or maple syrup
- 1 teaspoon cinnamon
- 2 cups almond milk
- 2 eggs

DIRECTIONS

1. Preheat oven to 375°F (190°C). Grease a baking dish.
2. Combine oats, walnuts, pears, honey, cinnamon, almond milk, and eggs.
3. Pour into dish and bake for 35 minutes.

Nutritional Information per serving: Calories: 240 | Total Fat: 8g | Saturated Fat: 1g | Trans Fat: 0g | Polyunsaturated Fat: 3g | Monounsaturated Fat: 3g | Cholesterol: 62mg | Sodium: 70mg | Carbohydrates: 36g | Fiber: 5g | Sugars: 15g | Protein: 8g

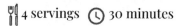

Savory Quinoa and Vegetable Breakfast Bowls

🍴 4 servings 🕐 30 minutes

INGREDIENTS
- 1 cup quinoa, rinsed
- 2 cups water
- 1 zucchini, diced
- 1 bell pepper, diced
- 1/2 onion, diced
- 1 tablespoon olive oil
- 1/4 cup grated Parmesan cheese
- Salt and pepper to taste

DIRECTIONS
1. Cook quinoa in water as per package instructions.
2. Sauté zucchini, bell pepper, and onion in olive oil.
3. Mix vegetables with cooked quinoa, add Parmesan, salt, and pepper.

Nutritional Information per serving: Calories: 280 | Total Fat: 9g | Saturated Fat: 2g | Trans Fat: 0g | Polyunsaturated Fat: 1g | Monounsaturated Fat: 5g | Cholesterol: 4mg | Sodium: 120mg | Carbohydrates: 39g | Fiber: 5g | Sugars: 3g | Protein: 11g

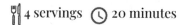

Whole Grain Waffles with Sliced Peaches and Honey

🍴 4 servings 🕐 20 minutes

INGREDIENTS
- 2 cups whole grain waffle mix
- 1 3/4 cups water or milk
- 1 egg
- 2 peaches, sliced
- Honey for drizzling

DIRECTIONS
1. Prepare waffle batter with mix, water/milk, and egg.
2. Cook waffles in a waffle iron.
3. Serve with sliced peaches and a drizzle of honey.

Nutritional Information per serving: Calories: 290 | Total Fat: 5g | Saturated Fat: 1g | Trans Fat: 0g | Polyunsaturated Fat: 2g | Monounsaturated Fat: 1g | Cholesterol: 47mg | Sodium: 480mg | Carbohydrates: 53g | Fiber: 8g | Sugars: 15g | Protein: 10g

Mediterranean Scramble with Tomatoes, Olives, and Feta

🍴 4 servings 🕐 15 minutes

INGREDIENTS
- 6 eggs, beaten
- 1 cup cherry tomatoes, halved
- 1/2 cup Kalamata olives, chopped
- 1/2 cup feta cheese, crumbled
- 1 tablespoon olive oil
- Salt and pepper to taste
- Fresh basil for garnish

DIRECTIONS
1. Heat olive oil in a skillet. Add tomatoes and olives, cook for a few minutes.
2. Pour beaten eggs over vegetables. Cook, stirring, until eggs are set.
3. Stir in feta cheese. Season with salt and pepper.
4. Garnish with fresh basil before serving.

Nutritional Information per serving: Calories: 230 | Total Fat: 18g | Saturated Fat: 6g | Trans Fat: 0g | Polyunsaturated Fat: 2g | Monounsaturated Fat: 9g | Cholesterol: 279mg | Sodium: 610mg | Carbohydrates: 6g | Fiber: 1g | Sugars: 3g | Protein: 13g

Multigrain Porridge with Dates and Spices

🍴 4 servings 🕐 20 minutes

INGREDIENTS
- 1/2 cup rolled oats
- 1/4 cup quinoa
- 1/4 cup millet
- 4 cups water or milk
- 1/2 cup dates, chopped
- 1 teaspoon cinnamon
- 1/2 teaspoon nutmeg
- Honey or maple syrup (optional)

DIRECTIONS
1. Combine oats, quinoa, millet, and water/milk in a pot.
2. Bring to a boil, then simmer for 15 minutes.
3. Stir in dates, cinnamon, and nutmeg.
4. Sweeten with honey or maple syrup if desired.

Nutritional Information per serving: Calories: 210 | Total Fat: 3g | Saturated Fat: 0.5g | Trans Fat: 0g | Polyunsaturated Fat: 1g | Monounsaturated Fat: 1g | Cholesterol: 0mg | Sodium: 10mg | Carbohydrates: 40g | Fiber: 5g | Sugars: 10g | Protein: 6g

Apple Cinnamon Breakfast Barley

🍴 4 servings 🕐 35 minutes

INGREDIENTS

- 1 cup barley
- 3 cups water
- 2 apples, diced
- 1 teaspoon cinnamon
- 1/4 teaspoon nutmeg
- Honey or maple syrup (optional)

DIRECTIONS

1. Cook barley in water as per package instructions.
2. In the last 10 minutes of cooking, add diced apples, cinnamon, and nutmeg.
3. Sweeten with honey or maple syrup if desired.

Nutritional Information per serving: Calories: 220 | Total Fat: 1g | Saturated Fat: 0g | Trans Fat: 0g | Polyunsaturated Fat: 0.5g | Monounsaturated Fat: 0.5g | Cholesterol: 0mg | Sodium: 10mg | Carbohydrates: 50g | Fiber: 9g | Sugars: 10g | Protein: 5g

Zucchini and Carrot Breakfast Muffins

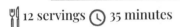 12 servings ⏱ 35 minutes

INGREDIENTS

- 1 cup whole wheat flour
- 1/2 cup oat flour
- 1/4 cup honey or maple syrup
- 2 teaspoons baking powder
- 1/2 teaspoon baking soda
- 1/4 teaspoon salt
- 1 cup grated zucchini
- 1 cup grated carrot
- 2 eggs
- 1/2 cup unsweetened applesauce
- 1/4 cup olive oil
- 1 teaspoon vanilla extract

DIRECTIONS

1. Preheat the oven to 350°F (175°C). Line a muffin tin with paper liners.
2. Mix both flours, baking powder, baking soda, and salt.
3. Stir in zucchini and carrot.
4. In another bowl, beat eggs with honey, applesauce, olive oil, and vanilla.
5. Combine wet and dry ingredients.
6. Pour into muffin tins and bake for 20 minutes.

Nutritional Information per serving: Calories: 180 | Total Fat: 6g | Saturated Fat: 1g | Trans Fat: 0g | Polyunsaturated Fat: 1g | Monounsaturated Fat: 3g | Cholesterol: 31mg | Sodium: 150mg | Carbohydrates: 28g | Fiber: 3g | Sugars: 10g | Protein: 4g

Warm Millet Cereal with Cinnamon Apples

🍴 4 servings ⏱ 25 minutes

INGREDIENTS

- 1 cup millet
- 3 cups water or milk
- 2 apples, diced
- 1 teaspoon cinnamon
- Honey or maple syrup (optional)

DIRECTIONS

1. Cook millet in water/milk as per package instructions.
2. In the last 5 minutes, add diced apples and cinnamon.
3. Sweeten with honey or maple syrup if desired.

Nutritional Information per serving: Calories: 235 | Total Fat: 3g | Saturated Fat: 0.5g | Trans Fat: 0g | Polyunsaturated Fat: 1g | Monounsaturated Fat: 1g | Cholesterol: 0mg | Sodium: 15mg | Carbohydrates: 47g | Fiber: 6g | Sugars: 12g | Protein: 6g

Tomato and Basil Breakfast Bruschetta

🍴 4 servings ⏱ 15 minutes

INGREDIENTS

- 4 slices whole grain bread
- 2 tomatoes, diced
- 1/4 cup fresh basil, chopped
- 1 tablespoon olive oil
- Salt and pepper to taste

DIRECTIONS

1. Toast the bread slices.
2. Mix tomatoes with basil, olive oil, salt, and pepper.
3. Top each slice of toast with the tomato mixture.

Nutritional Information per serving: Calories: 120 | Total Fat: 4g | Saturated Fat: 0.5g | Trans Fat: 0g | Polyunsaturated Fat: 0.5g | Monounsaturated Fat: 2.5g | Cholesterol: 0mg | Sodium: 180mg | Carbohydrates: 18g | Fiber: 3g | Sugars: 3g | Protein: 4g

Peanut Butter and Strawberry Chia Jam on Sprouted Grain Bread

🍴 2 servings ⏱ 10 minutes

INGREDIENTS
- 4 slices sprouted grain bread
- 1/4 cup natural peanut butter
- 1/2 cup strawberries, mashed
- 1 tablespoon chia seeds
- 1 tablespoon honey or maple syrup (optional)

DIRECTIONS
1. Toast the bread slices.
2. Mix mashed strawberries with chia seeds and honey/maple syrup if using. Let sit for 10 minutes.
3. Spread peanut butter on toast, then top with chia jam.

Nutritional Information per serving: Calories: 380 | Total Fat: 18g | Saturated Fat: 3g | Trans Fat: 0g | Polyunsaturated Fat: 5g | Monounsaturated Fat: 8g | Cholesterol: 0mg | Sodium: 300mg | Carbohydrates: 45g | Fiber: 9g | Sugars: 12g | Protein: 15g

Veggie and Herb Breakfast Polenta

🍴 4 servings 🕐 20 minutes

INGREDIENTS
- 1 cup polenta (cornmeal)
- 4 cups water or vegetable broth
- 1 zucchini, diced
- 1 bell pepper, diced
- 1/2 onion, diced
- 1/4 cup fresh herbs (parsley, thyme)
- 1 tablespoon olive oil
- Salt and pepper to taste

DIRECTIONS
1. Cook polenta in water/broth as per package instructions.
2. Sauté zucchini, bell pepper, and onion in olive oil.
3. Stir vegetables and herbs into cooked polenta.
4. Season with salt and pepper to taste.

Nutritional Information per serving: Calories: 210 | Total Fat: 4g | Saturated Fat: 0.5g | Trans Fat: 0g | Polyunsaturated Fat: 1g | Monounsaturated Fat: 2.5g | Cholesterol: 0mg | Sodium: 480mg | Carbohydrates: 37g | Fiber: 4g | Sugars: 3g | Protein: 5g

Pumpkin Spice Protein Pancakes (Made with Almond Flour)

🍴 4 servings 🕐 20 minutes

INGREDIENTS
- 1 cup almond flour
- 2 scoops vanilla protein powder
- 1/2 cup canned pumpkin puree

- 1 teaspoon pumpkin pie spice
- 2 eggs
- 1/4 cup almond milk
- 1 tablespoon maple syrup (optional)

DIRECTIONS
1. Mix almond flour, protein powder, and pumpkin pie spice.
2. Stir in pumpkin puree, eggs, almond milk, and maple syrup if using.
3. Cook pancakes on a non-stick skillet over medium heat.
4. Serve warm.

Nutritional Information per serving: Calories: 280 | Total Fat: 16g | Saturated Fat: 2g | Trans Fat: 0g | Polyunsaturated Fat: 3g | Monounsaturated Fat: 9g | Cholesterol: 93mg | Sodium: 70mg | Carbohydrates: 18g | Fiber: 5g | Sugars: 7g | Protein: 17g

Quinoa and Berry Breakfast Bowl

🍴 4 servings 🕐 25 minutes

INGREDIENTS
- 1/2 cup quinoa, rinsed and drained
- 1 cup water
- 1 cup mixed berries (strawberries, blueberries, raspberries)
- 2 tablespoons chopped almonds
- 1 tablespoon honey
- 1/2 teaspoon vanilla extract
- 1/2 cup Greek yogurt (low-fat or fat-free)

DIRECTIONS
1. In a small saucepan, bring 1 cup of water to a boil. Add the quinoa, reduce heat to low, cover, and simmer for 15 minutes or until the water is absorbed and quinoa is tender.
2. Fluff the cooked quinoa with a fork and let it cool for a few minutes.
3. In serving bowls, layer the cooked quinoa, mixed berries, and chopped almonds.
4. Drizzle honey over the top and add a splash of vanilla extract.
5. Top each bowl with a dollop of Greek yogurt.
6. Serve immediately and enjoy your nutritious and delicious quinoa and berry breakfast bowl.

Nutritional Information per serving: Calories: 250 | Total Fat: 6g | Saturated Fat: 0.5g | Trans Fat: 0g | Polyunsaturated Fat: 2g | Monounsaturated Fat: 3g | Cholesterol: 0mg | Sodium: 20mg | Carbohydrates: 45g | Fiber: 6g | Sugars: 15g | Protein: 8g

Sweet Potato and Kale Breakfast Hash

🍴 2 servings 🕐 35 minutes

INGREDIENTS

- 1 large sweet potato, peeled and diced
- 1 cup kale, chopped
- 1/2 red bell pepper, diced
- 1/2 onion, finely chopped
- 2 cloves garlic, minced
- 2 eggs
- 2 tablespoons olive oil
- Salt and pepper to taste

DIRECTIONS

1. In a large skillet, heat olive oil over medium heat. Add diced sweet potatoes and cook until they begin to soften, about 8-10 minutes.
2. Add chopped onion and red bell pepper to the skillet. Sauté until the vegetables are tender.
3. Stir in minced garlic and chopped kale. Cook for an additional 2-3 minutes until the kale is wilted.
4. Create two wells in the vegetable mixture and crack an egg into each well.
5. Cover the skillet and cook until the eggs are cooked to your liking, around 5 minutes for a slightly runny yolk.
6. Season with salt and pepper to taste.
7. Serve the sweet potato and kale hash with a side of hot sauce or salsa if desired.

Nutritional Information per serving: Calories: 320 | Total Fat: 18g | Saturated Fat: 3g | Trans Fat: 0g | Polyunsaturated Fat: 3g | Monounsaturated Fat: 11g | Cholesterol: 185mg | Sodium: 160mg | Carbohydrates: 35g | Fiber: 6g | Sugars: 7g | Protein: 10g

CHAPTER 3: LUNCH

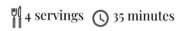
Grilled Chicken and Quinoa Salad

🍴 4 servings   🕐 35 minutes

INGREDIENTS
- 2 boneless, skinless chicken breasts
- 1 cup quinoa
- 2 cups water or chicken broth
- 1 bell pepper, diced
- 1 cucumber, diced
- 1/4 cup red onion, finely chopped
- 1/4 cup fresh parsley, chopped
- 2 tablespoons olive oil
- Juice of 1 lemon
- Salt and pepper to taste

DIRECTIONS
1. Cook quinoa in water or broth as per package instructions. Let it cool.
2. Grill chicken breasts until fully cooked, about 6-7 minutes per side. Let them rest, then slice.
3. In a large bowl, combine cooked quinoa, bell pepper, cucumber, red onion, and parsley.
4. Whisk together olive oil, lemon juice, salt, and pepper to make a dressing.
5. Toss the salad with the dressing, then top with sliced grilled chicken.

Nutritional Information per serving: Calories: 320 | Total Fat: 10g | Saturated Fat: 1.5g | Trans Fat: 0g | Polyunsaturated Fat: 1.5g | Monounsaturated Fat: 6g | Cholesterol: 50mg | Sodium: 150mg | Carbohydrates: 30g | Fiber: 4g | Sugars: 2g | Protein: 25g

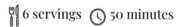
Lentil and Vegetable Soup

🍴 6 servings   🕐 50 minutes

INGREDIENTS
- 1 cup lentils, rinsed
- 1 onion, diced
- 2 carrots, diced
- 2 celery stalks, diced
- 2 garlic cloves, minced
- 1 can diced tomatoes
- 6 cups vegetable broth
- 1 teaspoon thyme
- 1 teaspoon rosemary
- Salt and pepper to taste
- 1 tablespoon olive oil

DIRECTIONS
1. In a large pot, heat olive oil over medium heat. Sauté onion, carrots, celery, and garlic until soft.
2. Add lentils, diced tomatoes, vegetable broth, thyme, and rosemary.
3. Bring to a boil, then reduce heat and simmer for 30-40 minutes, until lentils are tender.
4. Season with salt and pepper. Serve hot.

Nutritional Information per serving: Calories: 180 | Total Fat: 2.5g | Saturated Fat: 0.5g | Trans Fat: 0g | Polyunsaturated Fat: 0.5g | Monounsaturated Fat: 1.5g | Cholesterol: 0mg | Sodium: 480mg | Carbohydrates: 30g | Fiber: 10g | Sugars: 5g | Protein: 10g

Avocado and Turkey Lettuce Wraps

🍴 4 servings   🕐 10 minutes

INGREDIENTS
- 8 large lettuce leaves (e.g., romaine or butter lettuce)
- 8 ounces sliced turkey breast
- 1 ripe avocado, sliced
- 1 tomato, diced
- 1/4 red onion, thinly sliced
- Salt and pepper to taste

DIRECTIONS
1. Lay out lettuce leaves. Top each with turkey slices, avocado slices, diced tomato, and red onion.
2. Season with salt and pepper.
3. Fold in the sides of the lettuce and roll up to enclose the filling.

Nutritional Information per serving: Calories: 150 | Total Fat: 7g | Saturated Fat: 1g | Trans Fat: 0g | Polyunsaturated Fat: 1g | Monounsaturated Fat: 4g | Cholesterol: 25mg | Sodium: 450mg | Carbohydrates: 6g | Fiber: 4g | Sugars: 1g | Protein: 17g

Mediterranean Chickpea Salad

🍴 4 servings   🕐 15 minutes

INGREDIENTS

- 1 can chickpeas, drained and rinsed
- 1 cucumber, diced
- 1 bell pepper, diced
- 1/4 cup red onion, finely chopped
- 1/4 cup kalamata olives, sliced
- 1/4 cup feta cheese, crumbled
- 2 tablespoons olive oil
- Juice of 1 lemon
- 1 teaspoon dried oregano
- Salt and pepper to taste

DIRECTIONS

1. In a large bowl, combine chickpeas, cucumber, bell pepper, red onion, olives, and feta cheese.
2. In a small bowl, whisk together olive oil, lemon juice, oregano, salt, and pepper.
3. Pour dressing over salad and toss to combine.

Nutritional Information per serving: Calories: 250 | Total Fat: 12g | Saturated Fat: 3g | Trans Fat: 0g | Polyunsaturated Fat: 1g | Monounsaturated Fat: 7g | Cholesterol: 15mg | Sodium: 400mg | Carbohydrates: 28g | Fiber: 7g | Sugars: 5g | Protein: 9g

Baked Salmon with Steamed Broccoli

4 servings | 30 minutes

INGREDIENTS
- 4 salmon fillets (4 ounces each)
- 4 cups broccoli florets
- 2 tablespoons olive oil
- 1 lemon, sliced
- Salt and pepper to taste
- 1 teaspoon dill (optional)

DIRECTIONS

1. Preheat the oven to 375°F (190°C). Place salmon fillets on a baking sheet.
2. Drizzle salmon with 1 tablespoon olive oil and season with salt, pepper, and dill. Top with lemon slices.
3. Bake for 15-20 minutes or until salmon is cooked through.
4. Meanwhile, steam broccoli until tender.
5. Serve salmon with steamed broccoli on the side.

Nutritional Information per serving: Calories: 290 | Total Fat: 17g | Saturated Fat: 3g | Trans Fat: 0g | Polyunsaturated Fat: 5g | Monounsaturated Fat: 8g | Cholesterol: 60mg | Sodium: 200mg | Carbohydrates: 6g | Fiber: 3g | Sugars: 2g | Protein: 29g

Whole Wheat Pasta Primavera

4 servings | 35 minutes

INGREDIENTS
- 8 ounces whole wheat pasta
- 1 zucchini, sliced
- 1 yellow squash, sliced
- 1 bell pepper, chopped
- 1/2 cup cherry tomatoes, halved
- 2 cloves garlic, minced
- 1/4 cup olive oil
- Juice of 1 lemon
- Salt and pepper to taste
- 1/4 cup grated Parmesan cheese
- Fresh basil for garnish

DIRECTIONS

1. Cook pasta according to package instructions. Drain and set aside.
2. In a large skillet, heat olive oil over medium heat. Sauté garlic, zucchini, squash, and bell pepper until tender.
3. Add cherry tomatoes, cooked pasta, lemon juice, salt, and pepper. Toss to combine.
4. Serve topped with Parmesan cheese and fresh basil.

Nutritional Information per serving: Calories: 350 | Total Fat: 14g | Saturated Fat: 3g | Trans Fat: 0g | Polyunsaturated Fat: 2g | Monounsaturated Fat: 8g | Cholesterol: 5mg | Sodium: 200mg | Carbohydrates: 47g | Fiber: 8g | Sugars: 4g | Protein: 12g

Tuna Salad Stuffed Tomatoes

4 servings | 15 minutes

INGREDIENTS
- 4 large tomatoes
- 2 cans tuna in water, drained
- 1/4 cup low-fat Greek yogurt
- 1 celery stalk, finely chopped
- 2 tablespoons red onion, minced
- 1 tablespoon fresh dill, chopped
- Salt and pepper to taste
- Lemon wedges for serving

DIRECTIONS

1. Cut the tops off the tomatoes and scoop out the insides.
2. In a bowl, mix together tuna, Greek yogurt, celery, red onion, dill, salt, and pepper.

3. Stuff each tomato with the tuna salad.
4. Serve with lemon wedges.

Nutritional Information per serving: Calories: 180 | Total Fat: 2g | Saturated Fat: 0.5g | Trans Fat: 0g | Polyunsaturated Fat: 0.5g | Monounsaturated Fat: 0.5g | Cholesterol: 30mg | Sodium: 300mg | Carbohydrates: 10g | Fiber: 2g | Sugars: 6g | Protein: 27g

Veggie Hummus Wrap

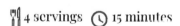 4 servings 🕐 10 minutes

INGREDIENTS
- 4 whole wheat tortillas
- 1 cup hummus
- 1 cucumber, thinly sliced
- 1 carrot, julienned
- 1 red bell pepper, thinly sliced
- 2 cups spinach leaves
- Salt and pepper to taste

DIRECTIONS
1. Spread hummus evenly over each tortilla.
2. Layer cucumber, carrot, bell pepper, and spinach on top of the hummus.
3. Season with salt and pepper.
4. Roll up the tortillas tightly, cut in half, and serve.

Nutritional Information per serving: Calories: 260 | Total Fat: 8g | Saturated Fat: 1g | Trans Fat: 0g | Polyunsaturated Fat: 2g | Monounsaturated Fat: 4g | Cholesterol: 0mg | Sodium: 480mg | Carbohydrates: 39g | Fiber: 7g | Sugars: 4g | Protein: 10g

Roasted Red Pepper and Spinach Panini

4 servings 🕐 15 minutes

INGREDIENTS
- 8 slices whole grain bread
- 1 cup roasted red peppers, sliced
- 2 cups fresh spinach
- 1/4 cup goat cheese, crumbled
- 1 tablespoon olive oil

DIRECTIONS
1. Assemble sandwiches with bread, roasted red peppers, spinach, and goat cheese.
2. Brush the outside of each sandwich with olive oil.
3. Grill in a panini press or on a skillet until golden brown and cheese is melted.

Nutritional Information per serving: Calories: 280 | Total Fat: 9g | Saturated Fat: 3g | Trans Fat: 0g | Polyunsaturated Fat: 1g | Monounsaturated Fat: 4g | Cholesterol: 10mg | Sodium: 500mg | Carbohydrates: 38g | Fiber: 6g | Sugars: 6g | Protein: 12g

Butternut Squash and Kale Stir-Fry

4 servings 🕐 35 minutes

INGREDIENTS
- 4 cups butternut squash, cubed
- 2 tablespoons olive oil
- 4 cups kale, chopped
- 2 cloves garlic, minced
- 1 teaspoon ground cumin
- Salt and pepper to taste
- 1/4 cup water or vegetable broth
- 2 tablespoons toasted pumpkin seeds

DIRECTIONS
1. Heat olive oil in a large skillet over medium heat. Add butternut squash and cook until slightly tender.
2. Add garlic, cumin, salt, and pepper. Cook for another minute.
3. Add kale and water or broth. Cover and cook until kale is wilted and squash is tender.
4. Serve garnished with toasted pumpkin seeds.

Nutritional Information per serving: Calories: 190 | Total Fat: 8g | Saturated Fat: 1g | Trans Fat: 0g | Polyunsaturated Fat: 1g | Monounsaturated Fat: 5g | Cholesterol: 0mg | Sodium: 50mg | Carbohydrates: 29g | Fiber: 6g | Sugars: 5g | Protein: 5g

Black Bean and Corn Salad

4 servings 🕐 10 minutes

INGREDIENTS
- 1 can black beans, drained and rinsed
- 1 cup corn kernels, fresh or frozen (thawed)
- 1 bell pepper, diced
- 1/4 cup red onion, finely chopped
- 1/4 cup cilantro, chopped
- Juice of 1 lime
- 2 tablespoons olive oil
- Salt and pepper to taste
- 1 avocado, diced

DIRECTIONS

1. In a large bowl, combine black beans, corn, bell pepper, red onion, and cilantro.
2. In a small bowl, whisk together lime juice, olive oil, salt, and pepper.
3. Pour the dressing over the salad and toss to combine.
4. Gently fold in the diced avocado before serving.

Nutritional Information per serving: Calories: 250 | Total Fat: 12g | Saturated Fat: 2g | Trans Fat: 0g | Polyunsaturated Fat: 1g | Monounsaturated Fat: 8g | Cholesterol: 0mg | Sodium: 200mg | Carbohydrates: 30g | Fiber: 10g | Sugars: 4g | Protein: 8g

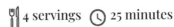

Grilled Vegetable and Goat Cheese Sandwich

🍴 4 servings 🕐 25 minutes

INGREDIENTS
- 8 slices whole-grain bread
- 1 zucchini, sliced lengthwise
- 1 red bell pepper, sliced
- 1 eggplant, sliced
- 4 ounces goat cheese
- 2 tablespoons olive oil
- Salt and pepper to taste
- 1 cup arugula or spinach

DIRECTIONS
1. Brush zucchini, bell pepper, and eggplant with olive oil and season with salt and pepper.
2. Grill vegetables until tender.
3. Spread goat cheese on 4 slices of bread. Top with grilled vegetables and arugula.
4. Place remaining bread slices on top and grill sandwiches until lightly toasted.

Nutritional Information per serving: Calories: 350 | Total Fat: 16g | Saturated Fat: 6g | Trans Fat: 0g | Polyunsaturated Fat: 2g | Monounsaturated Fat: 7g | Cholesterol: 13mg | Sodium: 400mg | Carbohydrates: 40g | Fiber: 9g | Sugars: 8g | Protein: 15g

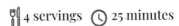

Cauliflower Rice Burrito Bowl

🍴 4 servings 🕐 25 minutes

INGREDIENTS
- 1 head cauliflower, riced
- 1 tablespoon olive oil
- 1 can black beans, drained and rinsed
- 1 cup corn kernels
- 1 teaspoon chili powder
- 1/2 teaspoon cumin

- Salt and pepper to taste
- 1 avocado, sliced
- 1/4 cup fresh salsa
- Lime wedges for serving

DIRECTIONS
1. Heat olive oil in a large skillet. Add cauliflower rice and cook for 5-7 minutes.
2. Add black beans, corn, chili powder, cumin, salt, and pepper. Cook until heated through.
3. Divide the mixture into bowls. Top with avocado slices and salsa.
4. Serve with lime wedges

Nutritional Information per serving: Calories: 280 | Total Fat: 11g | Saturated Fat: 1.5g | Trans Fat: 0g | Polyunsaturated Fat: 2g | Monounsaturated Fat: 6g | Cholesterol: 0mg | Sodium: 300mg | Carbohydrates: 40g | Fiber: 15g | Sugars: 6g | Protein: 11g

Shrimp and Avocado Salad

🍴 4 servings 🕐 20 minutes

INGREDIENTS
- 1 pound shrimp, peeled and deveined
- 2 tablespoons olive oil
- Salt and pepper to taste
- 4 cups mixed greens
- 1 avocado, sliced
- 1/4 cup red onion, thinly sliced
- 1/4 cup cilantro, chopped
- Juice of 1 lime
- 2 tablespoons extra virgin olive oil

DIRECTIONS
1. Heat olive oil in a skillet over medium-high heat. Add shrimp, season with salt and pepper, and cook until pink and opaque.
2. In a large bowl, toss mixed greens, avocado, red onion, and cilantro.
3. In a small bowl, whisk together lime juice and extra virgin olive oil, season with salt and pepper.
4. Add shrimp to the salad and drizzle with the dressing.

Nutritional Information per serving: Calories: 290 | Total Fat: 20g | Saturated Fat: 3g | Trans Fat: 0g | Polyunsaturated Fat: 3g | Monounsaturated Fat: 13g | Cholesterol: 143mg | Sodium: 470mg | Carbohydrates: 9g | Fiber: 5g | Sugars: 1g | Protein: 20g

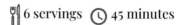

Sweet Potato and Black Bean Chili

🍴 6 servings 🕐 45 minutes

INGREDIENTS
- 2 tablespoons olive oil
- 1 onion, chopped
- 2 cloves garlic, minced
- 2 sweet potatoes, peeled and diced
- 1 can black beans, drained and rinsed
- 1 can diced tomatoes
- 2 tablespoons chili powder
- 1 teaspoon cumin
- 4 cups vegetable broth
- Salt and pepper to taste
- Fresh cilantro for garnish

DIRECTIONS
1. Heat olive oil in a large pot. Add onion and garlic, sauté until soft.
2. Add sweet potatoes, black beans, tomatoes, chili powder, and cumin. Stir to combine.
3. Pour in vegetable broth, bring to a boil, then reduce heat and simmer for 25-30 minutes, until sweet potatoes are tender.
4. Season with salt and pepper. Garnish with cilantro before serving.

Nutritional Information per serving: Calories: 220 | Total Fat: 5g | Saturated Fat: 1g | Trans Fat: 0g | Polyunsaturated Fat: 1g | Monounsaturated Fat: 3g | Cholesterol: 0mg | Sodium: 700mg | Carbohydrates: 37g | Fiber: 10g | Sugars: 7g | Protein: 8g

Rainbow Veggie and Quinoa Bowl

🍴 4 servings 🕐 40 minutes

INGREDIENTS
- 1 cup quinoa, rinsed
- 2 cups water
- 1/2 cup red cabbage, shredded
- 1/2 cup carrots, julienned
- 1/2 cup bell pepper, sliced
- 1/2 cup cucumber, sliced
- 1 avocado, sliced
- 1/4 cup sunflower seeds
- Salt and pepper to taste
- Dressing of choice (e.g., lemon vinaigrette)

DIRECTIONS
1. Cook quinoa in water according to package instructions.

2. Assemble bowls with cooked quinoa, red cabbage, carrots, bell pepper, cucumber, and avocado.
3. Sprinkle with sunflower seeds, season with salt and pepper.
4. Drizzle with your choice of dressing before serving.

Nutritional Information per serving: Calories: 310 | Total Fat: 15g | Saturated Fat: 2g | Trans Fat: 0g | Polyunsaturated Fat: 4g | Monounsaturated Fat: 8g | Cholesterol: 0mg | Sodium: 30mg | Carbohydrates: 39g | Fiber: 9g | Sugars: 4g | Protein: 10g

Spinach and Feta Stuffed Chicken Breast

🍴 4 servings 🕐 45 minutes

INGREDIENTS
- 4 boneless, skinless chicken breasts
- 2 cups fresh spinach, chopped
- 1/2 cup feta cheese, crumbled
- 2 cloves garlic, minced
- 1 tablespoon olive oil
- Salt and pepper to taste
- 1 teaspoon dried oregano
- 1 lemon, sliced for garnish

DIRECTIONS
1. Preheat the oven to 375°F (190°C).
2. In a skillet, heat olive oil over medium heat. Sauté garlic for 1 minute. Add spinach and cook until wilted, about 3-4 minutes. Remove from heat and let cool slightly. Stir in feta cheese.
3. Make a pocket in each chicken breast by slicing along the side. Be careful not to cut all the way through.
4. Stuff each chicken breast with the spinach and feta mixture. Secure with toothpicks if needed.
5. Season the outside of the chicken breasts with salt, pepper, and oregano.
6. Place the stuffed chicken breasts in a baking dish. Bake for 25 minutes or until the chicken is cooked through and no longer pink in the center.
7. Serve hot, garnished with lemon slices.

Nutritional Information per serving: Calories: 280 | Total Fat: 13g | Saturated Fat: 4g | Trans Fat: 0g | Polyunsaturated Fat: 2g | Monounsaturated Fat: 6g | Cholesterol: 110mg | Sodium: 400mg | Carbohydrates: 3g | Fiber: 1g | Sugars: 1g | Protein: 37g

Asian-Style Tofu and Broccoli Stir-Fry

🍴 4 servings 🕐 25 minutes

INGREDIENTS

- 14 oz firm tofu, drained and cubed
- 4 cups broccoli florets
- 2 tablespoons sesame oil
- 2 cloves garlic, minced
- 1 tablespoon fresh ginger, grated
- 3 tablespoons low-sodium soy sauce
- 1 tablespoon honey or maple syrup
- 1 teaspoon cornstarch mixed with 2 tablespoons water
- Sesame seeds for garnish

DIRECTIONS

1. Heat sesame oil in a large skillet or wok over medium heat. Add garlic and ginger, sauté for 1 minute.
2. Add tofu and stir-fry until golden brown, about 5 minutes.
3. Add broccoli and continue to stir-fry until tender-crisp, about 3-4 minutes.
4. In a small bowl, whisk together soy sauce, honey/maple syrup, and cornstarch mixture. Pour over tofu and broccoli, stirring until the sauce thickens.
5. Garnish with sesame seeds and serve hot.

Nutritional Information per serving: Calories: 200 | Total Fat: 11g | Saturated Fat: 1.5g | Trans Fat: 0g | Polyunsaturated Fat: 5g | Monounsaturated Fat: 4g | Cholesterol: 0mg | Sodium: 450mg | Carbohydrates: 15g | Fiber: 3g | Sugars: 6g | Protein: 12g

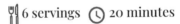

Turkey and Vegetable Meatloaf

🍴 6 servings   🕐 20 minutes

INGREDIENTS

- 1 lb ground turkey (lean)
- 1 cup zucchini, grated
- 1 cup carrots, grated
- 1 onion, finely chopped
- 2 cloves garlic, minced
- 1 egg, beaten
- 1/2 cup whole wheat breadcrumbs
- 1/4 cup ketchup
- 2 tablespoons Worcestershire sauce
- Salt and pepper to taste
- 1/4 cup fresh parsley, chopped

DIRECTIONS

1. Preheat oven to 375°F (190°C). Line a loaf pan with parchment paper.
2. In a large bowl, combine ground turkey, zucchini, carrots, onion, garlic, egg, breadcrumbs, half of the ketchup, Worcestershire sauce, salt, and pepper.
3. Press the mixture into the prepared loaf pan.

4. Spread the remaining ketchup over the top.
5. Bake for 1 hour or until cooked through.
6. Let it cool for 10 minutes before slicing. Garnish with fresh parsley.

Nutritional Information per serving: Calories: 220 | Total Fat: 10g | Saturated Fat: 2.5g | Trans Fat: 0g | Polyunsaturated Fat: 2.5g | Monounsaturated Fat: 4g | Cholesterol: 80mg | Sodium: 350mg | Carbohydrates: 15g | Fiber: 2g | Sugars: 6g | Protein: 20g

Greek Yogurt Chicken Salad

🍴 4 servings   🕐 15 minutes

INGREDIENTS

- 2 cups cooked chicken breast, shredded
- 1/2 cup Greek yogurt (non-fat)
- 1/4 cup celery, chopped
- 1/4 cup red grapes, halved
- 1/4 cup almonds, sliced
- 1 tablespoon lemon juice
- Salt and pepper to taste
- Fresh dill, chopped (optional)

DIRECTIONS

1. In a large bowl, combine shredded chicken, Greek yogurt, celery, grapes, and almonds.
2. Add lemon juice, salt, pepper, and dill if using. Mix well.
3. Serve chilled, on whole wheat bread or over a bed of greens.

Nutritional Information per serving: Calories: 180 | Total Fat: 4.5g | Saturated Fat: 0.5g | Trans Fat: 0g | Polyunsaturated Fat: 1g | Monounsaturated Fat: 2g | Cholesterol: 50mg | Sodium: 150mg | Carbohydrates: 8g | Fiber: 1g | Sugars: 5g | Protein: 27g

Zucchini Noodle Caprese

🍴 4 servings   🕐 15 minutes

INGREDIENTS

- 4 medium zucchini, spiralized
- 1 cup cherry tomatoes, halved
- 1/2 cup fresh mozzarella balls, halved
- 1/4 cup fresh basil, torn
- 2 tablespoons olive oil
- 1 tablespoon balsamic vinegar
- Salt and pepper to taste

DIRECTIONS

1. Place spiralized zucchini in a large bowl.
2. Add cherry tomatoes, mozzarella, and basil.

3.Drizzle with olive oil and balsamic vinegar.
4.Toss gently to combine. Season with salt and pepper.
5.Serve immediately or chill before serving.

Nutritional Information per serving: Calories: 150 | Total Fat: 11g | Saturated Fat: 3g | Trans Fat: 0g | Polyunsaturated Fat: 1g | Monounsaturated Fat: 6g | Cholesterol: 15mg | Sodium: 180mg | Carbohydrates: 8g | Fiber: 2g | Sugars: 5g | Protein: 7g

Moroccan Lentil and Vegetable Stew

🍴 4 servings 🕐 50 minutes

INGREDIENTS

- 1 cup lentils
- 1 onion, chopped
- 2 carrots, diced
- 2 celery stalks, diced
- 1 bell pepper, chopped
- 1 can diced tomatoes
- 4 cups vegetable broth
- 1 teaspoon cumin
- 1 teaspoon coriander
- 1/2 teaspoon cinnamon
- 2 tablespoons olive oil
- Salt and pepper to taste

DIRECTIONS

1.In a large pot, heat olive oil over medium heat. Add onion, carrots, celery, and bell pepper. Cook until softened.
2.Add lentils, tomatoes, vegetable broth, cumin, coriander, and cinnamon.
3.Bring to a boil, then reduce heat and simmer for 30-40 minutes.
4.Season with salt and pepper. Serve hot.

Nutritional Information per serving: Calories: 270 | Total Fat: 7g | Saturated Fat: 1g | Trans Fat: 0g | Polyunsaturated Fat: 1g | Monounsaturated Fat: 5g | Cholesterol: 0mg | Sodium: 300mg | Carbohydrates: 40g | Fiber: 15g | Sugars: 8g | Protein: 13g

Balsamic Grilled Vegetables with Arugula

🍴 4 servings 🕐 25 minutes

INGREDIENTS

- 2 zucchini, sliced
- 2 bell peppers, sliced
- 1 eggplant, sliced
- 1/4 cup balsamic vinegar

- 2 tablespoons olive oil
- 4 cups arugula
- Salt and pepper to taste

DIRECTIONS

1.Preheat grill to medium-high heat.
2.In a bowl, toss vegetables with balsamic vinegar, olive oil, salt, and pepper.
3.Grill vegetables until tender and charred.
4.Serve over a bed of arugula.

Nutritional Information per serving: Calories: 180 | Total Fat: 8g | Saturated Fat: 1g | Trans Fat: 0g | Polyunsaturated Fat: 1g | Monounsaturated Fat: 6g | Cholesterol: 0mg | Sodium: 75mg | Carbohydrates: 25g | Fiber: 9g | Sugars: 14g | Protein: 5g

Herb-Crusted Cod with Asparagus

🍴 4 servings 🕐 25 minutes

INGREDIENTS

- 4 cod fillets
- 1 bunch asparagus, trimmed
- 1/4 cup whole wheat breadcrumbs
- 1 tablespoon parsley, chopped
- 1 tablespoon dill, chopped
- 1 lemon, zested
- 2 tablespoons olive oil
- Salt and pepper to taste

DIRECTIONS

1.Preheat oven to 400°F (200°C).
2.Place cod and asparagus on a baking sheet. Drizzle with olive oil.
3.In a small bowl, combine breadcrumbs, parsley, dill, and lemon zest. Season with salt and pepper.
4.Press breadcrumb mixture onto cod fillets.
5.Bake for 15 minutes or until cod is cooked through and asparagus is tender.

Nutritional Information per serving: Calories: 210 | Total Fat: 7g | Saturated Fat: 1g | Trans Fat: 0g | Polyunsaturated Fat: 1g | Monounsaturated Fat: 5g | Cholesterol: 60mg | Sodium: 150mg | Carbohydrates: 9g | Fiber: 3g | Sugars: 2g | Protein: 28g

Tomato, Basil, and Mozzarella Zoodle Salad

🍴 4 servings 🕐 15 minutes

INGREDIENTS

- 4 medium zucchini, spiralized
- 1 cup cherry tomatoes, halved
- 1/2 cup fresh mozzarella balls, halved

- 1/4 cup fresh basil, torn
- 2 tablespoons olive oil
- 1 tablespoon balsamic vinegar
- Salt and pepper to taste

DIRECTIONS

1. In a large bowl, combine zoodles, cherry tomatoes, mozzarella, and basil.
2. In a small bowl, whisk together olive oil, balsamic vinegar, salt, and pepper.
3. Pour dressing over salad and toss to combine. Serve immediately.

Nutritional Information per serving: Calories: 150 | Total Fat: 11g | Saturated Fat: 3g | Trans Fat: 0g | Polyunsaturated Fat: 1g | Monounsaturated Fat: 6g | Cholesterol: 15mg | Sodium: 180mg | Carbohydrates: 8g | Fiber: 2g | Sugars: 5g | Protein: 7g

Spiced Chickpea and Sweet Potato Tacos

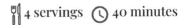

🍴 4 servings   🕐 40 minutes

INGREDIENTS

- 1 can chickpeas, drained and rinsed
- 2 sweet potatoes, diced
- 1 tablespoon olive oil
- 1 teaspoon paprika
- 1/2 teaspoon cumin
- 1/2 teaspoon garlic powder
- 8 corn tortillas
- 1 avocado, sliced
- 1/4 cup cilantro, chopped
- Lime wedges for serving

DIRECTIONS

1. Preheat oven to 400°F (200°C).
2. Toss sweet potatoes and chickpeas with olive oil, paprika, cumin, and garlic powder. Season with salt and pepper.
3. Spread on a baking sheet and roast for 20 minutes, stirring halfway through.
4. Warm tortillas in the oven or on a skillet.
5. Assemble tacos with sweet potato and chickpea mixture, avocado slices, and cilantro. Serve with lime wedges.

Nutritional Information per serving: Calories: 300 | Total Fat: 10g | Saturated Fat: 1.5g | Trans Fat: 0g | Polyunsaturated Fat: 2g | Monounsaturated Fat: 6g | Cholesterol: 0mg | Sodium: 200mg | Carbohydrates: 45g | Fiber: 10g | Sugars: 5g | Protein: 9g

Beetroot and Goat Cheese Salad

🍴 4 servings   🕐 15 minutes

INGREDIENTS

- 4 medium beetroots, cooked and sliced
- 2 cups mixed salad greens
- 1/2 cup goat cheese, crumbled
- 1/4 cup walnuts, chopped
- 2 tablespoons olive oil
- 1 tablespoon balsamic vinegar
- Salt and pepper to taste

DIRECTIONS

1. Arrange salad greens on plates.
2. Top with sliced beetroots, goat cheese, and walnuts.
3. In a small bowl, whisk together olive oil, balsamic vinegar, salt, and pepper.
4. Drizzle dressing over each salad.

Nutritional Information per serving: Calories: 200 | Total Fat: 15g | Saturated Fat: 4g | Trans Fat: 0g | Polyunsaturated Fat: 3g | Monounsaturated Fat: 7g | Cholesterol: 10mg | Sodium: 180mg | Carbohydrates: 10g | Fiber: 2g | Sugars: 7g | Protein: 6g

Eggplant and Chickpea Curry

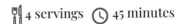

🍴 4 servings   🕐 45 minutes

INGREDIENTS

- 1 large eggplant, diced
- 1 can chickpeas, drained and rinsed
- 1 onion, chopped
- 2 cloves garlic, minced
- 1 can diced tomatoes
- 1 can coconut milk
- 1 tablespoon curry powder
- 1 teaspoon turmeric
- 1 teaspoon cumin
- 2 tablespoons olive oil
- Salt and pepper to taste
- Fresh cilantro for garnish

DIRECTIONS

1. Heat olive oil in a large pot over medium heat. Add onion and garlic, cook until soft.
2. Add eggplant and cook until slightly tender.
3. Stir in curry powder, turmeric, and cumin. Cook for 1 minute.
4. Add chickpeas, diced tomatoes, and coconut milk. Bring to a simmer and cook for 20 minutes.

5. Season with salt and pepper. Garnish with fresh cilantro.

Nutritional Information per serving: Calories: 350 | Total Fat: 22g | Saturated Fat: 13g | Trans Fat: 0g | Polyunsaturated Fat: 2g | Monounsaturated Fat: 6g | Cholesterol: 0mg | Sodium: 300mg | Carbohydrates: 33g | Fiber: 9g | Sugars: 9g | Protein: 9g

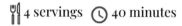

Pesto Chicken and Veggie Skewers

🍴 4 servings 🕐 40 minutes

INGREDIENTS
- 2 chicken breasts, cut into cubes
- 1 zucchini, sliced
- 1 red bell pepper, cut into squares
- 1 yellow bell pepper, cut into squares
- 1/2 cup homemade or store-bought pesto
- Salt and pepper to taste
- Wooden or metal skewers

DIRECTIONS
1. Preheat grill to medium-high heat.
2. Thread chicken, zucchini, and bell peppers onto skewers.
3. Brush skewers with pesto and season with salt and pepper.
4. Grill for 10 minutes, turning occasionally, until chicken is cooked through.
5. Serve hot.

Nutritional Information per serving: Calories: 250 | Total Fat: 10g | Saturated Fat: 2g | Trans Fat: 0g | Polyunsaturated Fat: 2g | Monounsaturated Fat: 5g | Cholesterol: 65mg | Sodium: 200mg | Carbohydrates: 10g | Fiber: 2g | Sugars: 4g | Protein: 28g

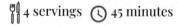

Quinoa Stuffed Bell Peppers

🍴 4 servings 🕐 45 minutes

INGREDIENTS
- 4 large bell peppers, tops removed and seeded
- 1 cup quinoa, cooked
- 1 can black beans, drained and rinsed
- 1 cup corn kernels
- 1/2 cup tomato sauce
- 1 teaspoon cumin
- 1 teaspoon paprika
- 1/2 cup shredded low-fat cheese
- Salt and pepper to taste

DIRECTIONS

1. Preheat oven to 350°F (175°C).
2. In a bowl, mix together quinoa, black beans, corn, tomato sauce, cumin, and paprika. Season with salt and pepper.
3. Stuff each bell pepper with the quinoa mixture.
4. Place in a baking dish and cover with foil.
5. Bake for 25 minutes, then remove foil, top with cheese, and bake for another 5 minutes.
6. Serve warm.

Nutritional Information per serving: Calories: 320 | Total Fat: 5g | Saturated Fat: 2g | Trans Fat: 0g | Polyunsaturated Fat: 1g | Monounsaturated Fat: 1g | Cholesterol: 10mg | Sodium: 400mg | Carbohydrates: 55g | Fiber: 10g | Sugars: 8g | Protein: 16g

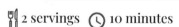

Broccoli and Almond Soup

🍴 4 servings 🕐 30 minutes

INGREDIENTS
- 4 cups broccoli florets
- 1 onion, chopped
- 2 cloves garlic, minced
- 4 cups vegetable broth
- 1/2 cup almonds, toasted
- 1 tablespoon olive oil
- Salt and pepper to taste

DIRECTIONS
1. In a large pot, heat olive oil over medium heat. Add onion and garlic, sauté until soft.
2. Add broccoli and vegetable broth. Bring to a boil, then reduce heat and simmer for 15 minutes.
3. Add almonds to the soup.
4. Blend soup using an immersion blender or in batches in a blender until smooth.
5. Season with salt and pepper. Serve hot.

Nutritional Information per serving: Calories: 180 | Total Fat: 11g | Saturated Fat: 1g | Trans Fat: 0g | Polyunsaturated Fat: 3g | Monounsaturated Fat: 6g | Cholesterol: 0mg | Sodium: 950mg | Carbohydrates: 16g | Fiber: 5g | Sugars: 4g | Protein: 7g

Smoked Salmon and Cucumber Sandwich

🍴 2 servings 🕐 10 minutes

INGREDIENTS
- 4 slices whole grain bread
- 4 ounces smoked salmon
- 1/2 cucumber, thinly sliced
- 1/4 cup low-fat cream cheese
- 1 tablespoon fresh dill, chopped

- Salt and pepper to taste

DIRECTIONS

1. Spread cream cheese evenly on two slices of bread.
2. Place smoked salmon over the cream cheese.
3. Add cucumber slices on top of the salmon.
4. Sprinkle with fresh dill, salt, and pepper.
5. Top with the remaining bread slices to make two sandwiches.
6. Cut in half and serve.

Nutritional Information per serving: Calories: 320 | Total Fat: 12g | Saturated Fat: 3g | Trans Fat: 0g | Polyunsaturated Fat: 3g | Monounsaturated Fat: 5g | Cholesterol: 30mg | Sodium: 720mg | Carbohydrates: 32g | Fiber: 5g | Sugars: 5g | Protein: 22g

Stuffed Portobello Mushrooms

🍴 4 servings 🕐 35 minutes

INGREDIENTS

- 4 large Portobello mushrooms, stems removed
- 1 cup cooked quinoa
- 1/2 cup spinach, chopped
- 1/4 cup sun-dried tomatoes, chopped
- 1/4 cup feta cheese, crumbled
- 2 cloves garlic, minced
- 1 tablespoon olive oil
- Salt and pepper to taste
- Balsamic glaze for drizzling (optional)

DIRECTIONS

1. Preheat the oven to 375°F (190°C).
2. In a bowl, mix quinoa, spinach, sun-dried tomatoes, feta cheese, garlic, salt, and pepper.
3. Brush each mushroom cap with olive oil. Stuff with the quinoa mixture.
4. Place stuffed mushrooms on a baking sheet and bake for 20 minutes.
5. Drizzle with balsamic glaze before serving, if desired.

Nutritional Information per serving: Calories: 180 | Total Fat: 7g | Saturated Fat: 2g | Trans Fat: 0g | Polyunsaturated Fat: 1g | Monounsaturated Fat: 3g | Cholesterol: 10mg | Sodium: 200mg | Carbohydrates: 22g | Fiber: 4g | Sugars: 5g | Protein: 8g

Vegetable and Lentil Soup

🍴 6 servings 🕐 55 minutes

INGREDIENTS

- 1 cup lentils, rinsed
- 1 onion, diced
- 2 carrots, diced
- 2 celery stalks, diced
- 1 bell pepper, diced
- 3 cloves garlic, minced
- 1 can diced tomatoes
- 6 cups vegetable broth
- 2 teaspoons Italian seasoning
- 1 bay leaf
- 2 tablespoons olive oil
- Salt and pepper to taste
- Fresh parsley for garnish

DIRECTIONS

1. In a large pot, heat olive oil over medium heat. Sauté onion, carrots, celery, bell pepper, and garlic until softened.
2. Add lentils, diced tomatoes, vegetable broth, Italian seasoning, and bay leaf.
3. Bring to a boil, then reduce heat and simmer for 30-40 minutes, until lentils are tender.
4. Season with salt and pepper. Garnish with fresh parsley.
5. Serve hot.

Nutritional Information per serving: Calories: 210 | Total Fat: 5g | Saturated Fat: 1g | Trans Fat: 0g | Polyunsaturated Fat: 1g | Monounsaturated Fat: 3g | Cholesterol: 0mg | Sodium: 500mg | Carbohydrates: 32g | Fiber: 11g | Sugars: 7g | Protein: 11g

Barley and Roasted Vegetable Salad

🍴 4 servings 🕐 45 minutes

INGREDIENTS

- 1 cup barley
- 2 cups water
- 1 zucchini, diced
- 1 red bell pepper, diced
- 1 yellow bell pepper, diced
- 1 red onion, diced
- 2 tablespoons olive oil
- 1/4 cup balsamic vinegar
- Salt and pepper to taste
- Fresh basil, chopped for garnish

DIRECTIONS

1. Preheat the oven to 400°F (200°C).
2. Cook barley in water according to package instructions.
3. Toss zucchini, bell peppers, and onion with olive oil, salt, and pepper. Roast on a baking sheet for 20 minutes.
4. In a large bowl, combine cooked barley with

roasted vegetables.
5.Drizzle with balsamic vinegar and toss.
6.Garnish with fresh basil before serving.

Nutritional Information per serving: Calories: 280 |
Total Fat: 8g | Saturated Fat: 1g | Trans Fat: 0g |
Polyunsaturated Fat: 1g | Monounsaturated Fat: 5g |
Cholesterol: 0mg | Sodium: 50mg | Carbohydrates:
46g | Fiber: 9g | Sugars: 7g | Protein: 7g

CHAPTER 4: DINNER

Garlic Lemon Herb Chicken

🍴 4 servings 🕐 45 minutes

INGREDIENTS
- 4 boneless, skinless chicken breasts
- 4 cloves garlic, minced
- Juice of 1 lemon
- 2 tablespoons olive oil
- 1 tablespoon fresh rosemary, chopped
- 1 tablespoon fresh thyme, chopped
- Salt and pepper to taste

DIRECTIONS
1. Preheat the oven to 375°F (190°C).
2. In a bowl, combine garlic, lemon juice, olive oil, rosemary, thyme, salt, and pepper.
3. Place chicken in a baking dish and pour the mixture over it. Ensure each piece is well coated.
4. Bake for 30 minutes, or until the chicken is cooked through.
5. Serve with your choice of side, like steamed vegetables or a salad.

Nutritional Information per serving: Calories: 220 | Total Fat: 10g | Saturated Fat: 1.5g | Trans Fat: 0g | Polyunsaturated Fat: 1.5g | Monounsaturated Fat: 6.5g | Cholesterol: 70mg | Sodium: 200mg | Carbohydrates: 3g | Fiber: 0.5g | Sugars: 0.5g | Protein: 28g

Chickpea and Spinach Stew

🍴 4 servings 🕐 30 minutes

INGREDIENTS
- 1 can chickpeas, drained and rinsed
- 4 cups fresh spinach
- 1 onion, diced
- 2 cloves garlic, minced
- 1 can diced tomatoes
- 2 cups vegetable broth
- 1 teaspoon cumin
- 1 teaspoon paprika
- 2 tablespoons olive oil
- Salt and pepper to taste

DIRECTIONS
1. Heat olive oil in a large pot over medium heat. Sauté onion and garlic until translucent.
2. Add cumin and paprika, stir for a minute.
3. Add chickpeas, diced tomatoes, and vegetable broth. Bring to a simmer.
4. Stir in spinach and cook until wilted.
5. Season with salt and pepper. Serve hot.

Nutritional Information per serving: Calories: 210 | Total Fat: 7g | Saturated Fat: 1g | Trans Fat: 0g | Polyunsaturated Fat: 1g | Monounsaturated Fat: 5g | Cholesterol: 0mg | Sodium: 400mg | Carbohydrates: 29g | Fiber: 8g | Sugars: 6g | Protein: 9g

Grilled Trout with Herb Salad

🍴 4 servings 🕐 25 minutes

INGREDIENTS
- 4 trout fillets
- 1 lemon, sliced
- 2 tablespoons olive oil
- Salt and pepper to taste
- Herb Salad:
- 2 cups mixed herbs (parsley, dill, cilantro)
- 1 cup arugula
- Juice of 1 lemon
- 2 tablespoons olive oil
- Salt and pepper to taste

DIRECTIONS
1. Preheat grill to medium-high heat. Brush trout fillets with olive oil and season with salt and pepper.
2. Grill trout for 5 minutes on each side, or until cooked through. Place lemon slices on top during the last few minutes of grilling.
3. For the herb salad, combine herbs and arugula in a bowl. Dress with lemon juice, olive oil, salt, and pepper.
4. Serve grilled trout with the fresh herb salad.

Nutritional Information per serving: Calories: 290 | Total Fat: 17g | Saturated Fat: 3g | Trans Fat: 0g | Polyunsaturated Fat: 3g | Monounsaturated Fat: 10g | Cholesterol: 80mg | Sodium: 100mg | Carbohydrates: 6g | Fiber: 2g | Sugars: 2g | Protein: 28g

Baked Eggplant with Tomato and Feta

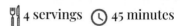 4 servings 🕐 45 minutes

INGREDIENTS

- 2 large eggplants, sliced into rounds
- 4 tomatoes, sliced
- 1/2 cup feta cheese, crumbled
- 3 tablespoons olive oil
- 2 cloves garlic, minced
- Fresh basil, torn
- Salt and pepper to taste

DIRECTIONS

1. Preheat oven to 400°F (200°C). Arrange eggplant slices on a baking sheet.
2. Brush each slice with olive oil and season with salt, pepper, and minced garlic.
3. Bake for 15 minutes.
4. Top each eggplant round with a tomato slice and feta cheese. Return to the oven and bake for an additional 10 minutes.
5. Garnish with fresh basil before serving.

Nutritional Information per serving: Calories: 200 | Total Fat: 15g | Saturated Fat: 4g | Trans Fat: 0g | Polyunsaturated Fat: 1g | Monounsaturated Fat: 9g | Cholesterol: 15mg | Sodium: 300mg | Carbohydrates: 15g | Fiber: 6g | Sugars: 9g | Protein: 5g

Roasted Red Pepper and Lentil Soup

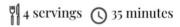 4 servings 🕐 35 minutes

INGREDIENTS

- 1 cup red lentils, rinsed
- 2 roasted red peppers, chopped
- 1 onion, diced
- 2 cloves garlic, minced
- 4 cups vegetable broth
- 1 teaspoon smoked paprika
- 2 tablespoons olive oil
- Salt and pepper to taste
- Fresh parsley for garnish

DIRECTIONS

1. Heat olive oil in a large pot over medium heat. Sauté onion and garlic until soft.
2. Add red lentils, roasted red peppers, smoked paprika, and vegetable broth.
3. Bring to a boil, then reduce heat and simmer for 20 minutes, or until lentils are tender.

4. Blend the soup using an immersion blender or transfer to a blender in batches until smooth.
5. Season with salt and pepper. Garnish with fresh parsley.
6. Serve hot.

Nutritional Information per serving: Calories: 230 | Total Fat: 7g | Saturated Fat: 1g | Trans Fat: 0g | Polyunsaturated Fat: 1g | Monounsaturated Fat: 5g | Cholesterol: 0mg | Sodium: 200mg | Carbohydrates: 33g | Fiber: 15g | Sugars: 4g | Protein: 11g

Stuffed Acorn Squash with Quinoa and Kale

🍴 4 servings 🕐 55 minutes

INGREDIENTS

- 2 acorn squashes, halved and seeded
- 1 cup quinoa, cooked
- 2 cups kale, chopped
- 1/4 cup dried cranberries
- 1/4 cup walnuts, chopped
- 2 tablespoons olive oil
- 1 teaspoon cinnamon
- Salt and pepper to taste

DIRECTIONS

1. Preheat oven to 375°F (190°C). Place acorn squash halves on a baking sheet, cut-side up. Brush with olive oil and sprinkle with cinnamon, salt, and pepper.
2. Roast for 25-30 minutes, until tender.
3. In a bowl, mix together cooked quinoa, kale, cranberries, and walnuts.
4. Once the squash is roasted, fill each half with the quinoa mixture.
5. Return to the oven and bake for an additional 10 minutes.
6. Serve warm.

Nutritional Information per serving: Calories: 330 | Total Fat: 12g | Saturated Fat: 1.5g | Trans Fat: 0g | Polyunsaturated Fat: 3.5g | Monounsaturated Fat: 6g | Cholesterol: 0mg | Sodium: 100mg | Carbohydrates: 53g | Fiber: 8g | Sugars: 9g | Protein: 8g

Rosemary Lemon Baked Cod

🍴 4 servings 🕐 25 minutes

INGREDIENTS

- 4 cod fillets
- Juice and zest of 1 lemon

- 2 tablespoons olive oil
- 2 cloves garlic, minced
- 1 tablespoon fresh rosemary, chopped
- Salt and pepper to taste

DIRECTIONS

1. Preheat the oven to 400°F (200°C).
2. In a small bowl, mix together lemon juice and zest, olive oil, garlic, and rosemary.
3. Place cod fillets in a baking dish. Season with salt and pepper.
4. Pour the lemon rosemary mixture over the cod.
5. Bake for 12-15 minutes, or until the fish flakes easily with a fork.
6. Serve with a side of steamed vegetables or a salad.

Nutritional Information per serving: Calories: 180 | Total Fat: 7g | Saturated Fat: 1g | Trans Fat: 0g | Polyunsaturated Fat: 1g | Monounsaturated Fat: 5g | Cholesterol: 60mg | Sodium: 70mg | Carbohydrates: 2g | Fiber: 0.5g | Sugars: 0.5g | Protein: 27g

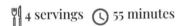

Mushroom and Barley Soup

🍴 4 servings 🕐 55 minutes

INGREDIENTS

- 1 cup pearl barley
- 1 onion, diced
- 2 carrots, diced
- 2 celery stalks, diced
- 3 cups mushrooms, sliced
- 6 cups vegetable broth
- 2 cloves garlic, minced
- 2 tablespoons olive oil
- 1 teaspoon thyme
- Salt and pepper to taste

DIRECTIONS

1. Heat olive oil in a large pot over medium heat. Sauté onion, carrots, celery, and garlic until soft.
2. Add mushrooms and thyme. Cook until mushrooms are tender.
3. Stir in barley and vegetable broth. Bring to a boil.
4. Reduce heat, cover, and simmer for 30-40 minutes, or until barley is tender.
5. Season with salt and pepper. Serve hot.

Nutritional Information per serving: Calories: 210 | Total Fat: 5g | Saturated Fat: 0.7g | Trans Fat: 0g | Polyunsaturated Fat: 0.7g | Monounsaturated Fat: 3.3g | Cholesterol: 0mg | Sodium: 300mg | Carbohydrates: 37g | Fiber: 8g | Sugars: 5g | Protein: 6g

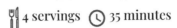

Orange Glazed Salmon with Asparagus

🍴 4 servings 🕐 35 minutes

INGREDIENTS

- 4 salmon fillets
- 1 bunch asparagus, trimmed
- Juice and zest of 1 orange
- 2 tablespoons honey
- 2 tablespoons soy sauce
- 1 clove garlic, minced
- 1 tablespoon ginger, grated
- 2 tablespoons olive oil
- Salt and pepper to taste

DIRECTIONS

1. Preheat the oven to 400°F (200°C).
2. In a small bowl, whisk together orange juice and zest, honey, soy sauce, garlic, and ginger.
3. Place salmon fillets and asparagus on a baking sheet. Drizzle with olive oil and season with salt and pepper.
4. Pour the orange glaze over the salmon.
5. Bake for 15-20 minutes, or until salmon is cooked through and asparagus is tender.
6. Serve immediately.

Nutritional Information per serving: Calories: 330 | Total Fat: 16g | Saturated Fat: 2.5g | Trans Fat: 0g | Polyunsaturated Fat: 4g | Monounsaturated Fat: 8g | Cholesterol: 70mg | Sodium: 320mg | Carbohydrates: 15g | Fiber: 2g | Sugars: 12g | Protein: 31g

Turmeric Cauliflower and Chickpea Curry

🍴 4 servings 🕐 45 minutes

INGREDIENTS

- 1 head cauliflower, cut into florets
- 1 can chickpeas, drained and rinsed
- 1 onion, diced
- 2 cloves garlic, minced
- 1 can coconut milk
- 2 tablespoons curry powder
- 1 teaspoon turmeric
- 1 teaspoon cumin
- 2 tablespoons olive oil
- Salt and pepper to taste
- Fresh cilantro for garnish

DIRECTIONS

1. Heat olive oil in a large pot over medium heat. Sauté onion and garlic until translucent.
2. Add curry powder, turmeric, and cumin. Cook for 1 minute, stirring constantly.
3. Add cauliflower and chickpeas. Stir to coat with spices.
4. Pour in coconut milk and bring to a simmer. Cover and cook for 20-25 minutes, or until cauliflower is tender.
5. Season with salt and pepper. Garnish with fresh cilantro.
6. Serve with brown rice or naan bread.

Nutritional Information per serving: Calories: 330 | Total Fat: 20g | Saturated Fat: 14g | Trans Fat: 0g | Polyunsaturated Fat: 2g | Monounsaturated Fat: 4g | Cholesterol: 0mg | Sodium: 300mg | Carbohydrates: 30g | Fiber: 8g | Sugars: 6g | Protein: 9g

Baked Tilapia with Mango Salsa

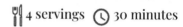 4 servings · 30 minutes

INGREDIENTS
- 4 tilapia fillets
- 2 mangos, diced
- 1 red bell pepper, diced
- 1/4 cup red onion, finely chopped
- 1/4 cup fresh cilantro, chopped
- Juice of 1 lime
- 1 tablespoon olive oil
- Salt and pepper to taste

DIRECTIONS
1. Preheat the oven to 400°F (200°C).
2. Place tilapia fillets on a baking sheet. Drizzle with olive oil and season with salt and pepper.
3. Bake for 12 minutes, or until fish flakes easily with a fork.
4. In a bowl, mix together mango, red bell pepper, red onion, cilantro, and lime juice to make the salsa.
5. Serve tilapia topped with mango salsa.

Nutritional Information per serving: Calories: 220 | Total Fat: 6g | Saturated Fat: 1g | Trans Fat: 0g | Polyunsaturated Fat: 1g | Monounsaturated Fat: 3g | Cholesterol: 55mg | Sodium: 100mg | Carbohydrates: 15g | Fiber: 2g | Sugars: 12g | Protein: 26g

Vegetable Paella with Brown Rice

4 servings · 55 minutes

INGREDIENTS
- 1 cup brown rice
- 4 cups vegetable broth
- 1 onion, diced
- 2 cloves garlic, minced
- 1 red bell pepper, sliced
- 1 yellow bell pepper, sliced
- 1 cup frozen peas
- 1 can artichoke hearts, drained and quartered
- 1 teaspoon saffron threads
- 1 teaspoon smoked paprika
- 2 tablespoons olive oil
- Salt and pepper to taste
- Fresh parsley for garnish
- Lemon wedges for serving

DIRECTIONS
1. Heat olive oil in a large skillet over medium heat. Sauté onion and garlic until soft.
2. Add bell peppers and cook for 5 minutes.
3. Stir in brown rice, saffron, smoked paprika, salt, and pepper. Cook for 2 minutes.
4. Add vegetable broth. Bring to a boil, then reduce heat and simmer, covered, for 30-35 minutes, or until rice is cooked.
5. Stir in peas and artichoke hearts. Cook for an additional 5 minutes.
6. Garnish with fresh parsley and serve with lemon wedges.

Nutritional Information per serving: Calories: 300 | Total Fat: 8g | Saturated Fat: 1g | Trans Fat: 0g | Polyunsaturated Fat: 1g | Monounsaturated Fat: 5g | Cholesterol: 0mg | Sodium: 950mg | Carbohydrates: 50g | Fiber: 6g | Sugars: 5g | Protein: 8g

Sesame Ginger Stir-Fry with Tofu

4 servings · 25 minutes

INGREDIENTS
- 14 oz firm tofu, cubed
- 2 cups broccoli florets
- 1 red bell pepper, sliced
- 1 carrot, sliced
- 2 tablespoons sesame oil
- 2 cloves garlic, minced
- 1 tablespoon fresh ginger, grated
- 3 tablespoons low-sodium soy sauce
- 1 tablespoon honey or maple syrup
- 1 tablespoon rice vinegar
- 1 teaspoon cornstarch mixed with 2 tablespoons water
- Sesame seeds for garnish
- Cooked brown rice for serving

DIRECTIONS

1. Heat sesame oil in a large skillet or wok over medium heat.
2. Add garlic, ginger, broccoli, bell pepper, and carrot. Stir-fry until vegetables are tender-crisp.
3. Add cubed tofu to the skillet. Cook until lightly browned.
4. In a small bowl, mix soy sauce, honey/maple syrup, rice vinegar, and cornstarch mixture.
5. Pour sauce over the stir-fry and cook until the sauce thickens.
6. Serve over brown rice and garnish with sesame seeds.

Nutritional Information per serving: Calories: 250 | Total Fat: 12g | Saturated Fat: 2g | Trans Fat: 0g | Polyunsaturated Fat: 5g | Monounsaturated Fat: 4g | Cholesterol: 0mg | Sodium: 320mg | Carbohydrates: 25g | Fiber: 4g | Sugars: 7g | Protein: 14g

Kale and White Bean Soup

🍴 4 servings 🕐 40 minutes

INGREDIENTS

- 1 onion, diced
- 2 carrots, diced
- 2 celery stalks, diced
- 3 cloves garlic, minced
- 4 cups kale, chopped
- 1 can white beans, drained and rinsed
- 6 cups vegetable broth
- 1 teaspoon thyme
- 2 tablespoons olive oil
- Salt and pepper to taste

DIRECTIONS

1. Heat olive oil in a large pot over medium heat.
2. Add onion, carrots, and celery. Sauté until softened.
3. Add garlic and thyme. Cook for another minute.
4. Add kale, white beans, and vegetable broth. Bring to a boil.
5. Reduce heat and simmer for 20 minutes.
6. Season with salt and pepper. Serve hot.

Nutritional Information per serving: Calories: 180 | Total Fat: 5g | Saturated Fat: 1g | Trans Fat: 0g | Polyunsaturated Fat: 1g | Monounsaturated Fat: 3g | Cholesterol: 0mg | Sodium: 400mg | Carbohydrates: 27g | Fiber: 6g | Sugars: 4g | Protein: 8g

Lemon Herb Roasted Chicken and Potatoes

🍴 4 servings 🕐 1 hour 15 minutes

INGREDIENTS

- 4 chicken breasts
- 4 medium potatoes, quartered
- Juice and zest of 2 lemons
- 3 tablespoons olive oil
- 2 cloves garlic, minced
- 1 tablespoon rosemary, chopped
- 1 tablespoon thyme, chopped
- Salt and pepper to taste

DIRECTIONS

1. Preheat the oven to 375°F (190°C).
2. In a large bowl, mix lemon juice and zest, olive oil, garlic, rosemary, thyme, salt, and pepper.
3. Add chicken and potatoes to the bowl. Toss to coat.
4. Place chicken and potatoes in a roasting pan.
5. Bake for 1 hour, or until chicken is cooked through and potatoes are tender.
6. Serve hot.

Nutritional Information per serving: Calories: 420 | Total Fat: 12g | Saturated Fat: 2g | Trans Fat: 0g | Polyunsaturated Fat: 2g | Monounsaturated Fat: 7g | Cholesterol: 95mg | Sodium: 200mg | Carbohydrates: 40g | Fiber: 5g | Sugars: 2g | Protein: 38g

Vegetarian Stuffed Zucchini Boats

🍴 4 servings 🕐 45 minutes

INGREDIENTS

- 4 medium zucchini, halved lengthwise
- 1 cup cooked quinoa
- 1 can black beans, drained and rinsed
- 1/2 cup corn kernels
- 1/2 cup tomato sauce
- 1 teaspoon cumin
- 1 teaspoon smoked paprika
- 1/2 cup shredded low-fat cheese
- Salt and pepper to taste
- Fresh cilantro for garnish

DIRECTIONS

1. Preheat the oven to 375°F (190°C).
2. Scoop out the centers of the zucchini halves to create boats.

3. In a bowl, mix quinoa, black beans, corn, tomato sauce, cumin, and smoked paprika. Season with salt and pepper.
4. Stuff the zucchini boats with the mixture.
5. Place in a baking dish and cover with foil.
6. Bake for 20 minutes. Remove foil, top with cheese, and bake for an additional 5 minutes.
7. Garnish with fresh cilantro before serving.

Nutritional Information per serving: Calories: 280 | Total Fat: 5g | Saturated Fat: 2g | Trans Fat: 0g | Polyunsaturated Fat: 1g | Monounsaturated Fat: 1g | Cholesterol: 10mg | Sodium: 400mg | Carbohydrates: 45g | Fiber: 12g | Sugars: 8g | Protein: 16g

Spicy Black Bean and Sweet Potato Chili

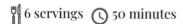 6 servings   50 minutes

INGREDIENTS

- 2 sweet potatoes, peeled and diced
- 2 cans black beans, drained and rinsed
- 1 onion, diced
- 2 cloves garlic, minced
- 1 can diced tomatoes
- 1 tablespoon chili powder
- 1 teaspoon cumin
- 1/2 teaspoon cayenne pepper (adjust to taste)
- 4 cups vegetable broth
- 2 tablespoons olive oil
- Salt and pepper to taste
- Fresh cilantro for garnish

DIRECTIONS

1. Heat olive oil in a large pot over medium heat.
2. Add onion and garlic, sauté until soft.
3. Add sweet potatoes, black beans, diced tomatoes, chili powder, cumin, cayenne pepper, and vegetable broth.
4. Bring to a boil, then reduce heat and simmer for 30 minutes, or until sweet potatoes are tender.
5. Season with salt and pepper. Garnish with fresh cilantro.
6. Serve hot.

Nutritional Information per serving: Calories: 230 | Total Fat: 5g | Saturated Fat: 1g | Trans Fat: 0g | Polyunsaturated Fat: 1g | Monounsaturated Fat: 3g | Cholesterol: 0mg | Sodium: 700mg | Carbohydrates: 40g | Fiber: 10g | Sugars: 7g | Protein: 10g

Baked Haddock with Spinach and Tomatoes

4 servings   30 minutes

INGREDIENTS

- 4 haddock fillets
- 4 cups spinach leaves
- 2 tomatoes, sliced
- 2 tablespoons olive oil
- 2 cloves garlic, minced
- 1 lemon, sliced
- Salt and pepper to taste

DIRECTIONS

1. Preheat the oven to 375°F (190°C).
2. Place haddock fillets in a baking dish.
3. Top each fillet with spinach, tomato slices, and minced garlic.
4. Drizzle with olive oil and season with salt and pepper.
5. Place lemon slices on top.
6. Bake for 20 minutes, or until fish is cooked through.
7. Serve hot.

Nutritional Information per serving: Calories: 200 | Total Fat: 7g | Saturated Fat: 1g | Trans Fat: 0g | Polyunsaturated Fat: 1g | Monounsaturated Fat: 5g | Cholesterol: 60mg | Sodium: 150mg | Carbohydrates: 6g | Fiber: 2g | Sugars: 2g | Protein: 27g

Butternut Squash Soup with Toasted Seeds

4 servings   55 minutes

INGREDIENTS

- 1 large butternut squash, peeled and cubed
- 1 onion, diced
- 3 cloves garlic, minced
- 4 cups vegetable broth
- 1 teaspoon cinnamon
- 1/2 teaspoon nutmeg
- 2 tablespoons olive oil
- Salt and pepper to taste
- Pumpkin seeds or squash seeds, toasted for garnish

DIRECTIONS

1. Heat olive oil in a large pot over medium heat. Sauté onion and garlic until translucent.
2. Add butternut squash, cinnamon, nutmeg, salt, and pepper. Cook for 5 minutes.

3. Pour in vegetable broth and bring to a boil. Reduce heat and simmer for 30 minutes, or until squash is tender.
4. Blend the soup using an immersion blender or in batches in a blender until smooth.
5. Serve hot, garnished with toasted pumpkin or squash seeds.

Nutritional Information per serving: Calories: 180 | Total Fat: 7g | Saturated Fat: 1g | Trans Fat: 0g | Polyunsaturated Fat: 1g | Monounsaturated Fat: 5g | Cholesterol: 0mg | Sodium: 480mg | Carbohydrates: 29g | Fiber: 5g | Sugars: 6g | Protein: 3g

Mediterranean Lentil Salad

🍴 4 servings   🕐 40 minutes

INGREDIENTS

- 1 cup green lentils
- 1 cucumber, diced
- 1 bell pepper, diced
- 1/2 red onion, finely chopped
- 1/2 cup kalamata olives, sliced
- 1/4 cup feta cheese, crumbled
- 1/4 cup fresh parsley, chopped
- 3 tablespoons olive oil
- 2 tablespoons red wine vinegar
- 1 teaspoon dried oregano
- Salt and pepper to taste

DIRECTIONS

1. Cook lentils according to package instructions. Drain and let cool.
2. In a large bowl, combine cooled lentils, cucumber, bell pepper, red onion, olives, feta cheese, and parsley.
3. In a small bowl, whisk together olive oil, red wine vinegar, oregano, salt, and pepper.
4. Pour dressing over the salad and toss to combine.
5. Serve chilled or at room temperature.

Nutritional Information per serving: Calories: 280 | Total Fat: 14g | Saturated Fat: 3g | Trans Fat: 0g | Polyunsaturated Fat: 1g | Monounsaturated Fat: 9g | Cholesterol: 10mg | Sodium: 320mg | Carbohydrates: 30g | Fiber: 12g | Sugars: 5g | Protein: 11g

Tandoori Grilled Vegetables

🍴 4 servings   🕐 30 minutes

INGREDIENTS

- 1 zucchini, sliced
- 1 bell pepper, sliced
- 1 eggplant, sliced
- 1 red onion, cut into wedges
- 2 tablespoons tandoori spice mix
- 3 tablespoons plain yogurt
- 2 tablespoons olive oil
- Salt to taste
- Fresh cilantro for garnish

DIRECTIONS

1. In a large bowl, mix yogurt, tandoori spice mix, olive oil, and salt.
2. Add vegetables to the bowl and toss to coat evenly.
3. Preheat grill to medium-high heat.
4. Grill vegetables for 5-7 minutes per side, or until charred and tender.
5. Garnish with fresh cilantro and serve.

Nutritional Information per serving: Calories: 120 | Total Fat: 7g | Saturated Fat: 1g | Trans Fat: 0g | Polyunsaturated Fat: 1g | Monounsaturated Fat: 5g | Cholesterol: 0mg | Sodium: 80mg | Carbohydrates: 13g | Fiber: 4g | Sugars: 8g | Protein: 3g

Pesto Stuffed Portobello Mushrooms

🍴 4 servings   🕐 35 minutes

INGREDIENTS

- 4 large Portobello mushrooms, stems removed
- 1/2 cup homemade or store-bought pesto
- 1/4 cup sun-dried tomatoes, chopped
- 1/4 cup feta cheese, crumbled
- 2 tablespoons olive oil
- Salt and pepper to taste

DIRECTIONS

1. Preheat the oven to 375°F (190°C).
2. Brush each mushroom cap with olive oil. Season with salt and pepper.
3. Spread pesto inside each mushroom cap.
4. Top with sun-dried tomatoes and feta cheese.
5. Bake for 20 minutes or until mushrooms are tender.
6. Serve warm.

Nutritional Information per serving: Calories: 200 | Total Fat: 16g | Saturated Fat: 3g | Trans Fat: 0g | Polyunsaturated Fat: 1g | Monounsaturated Fat: 11g | Cholesterol: 10mg | Sodium: 320mg | Carbohydrates: 9g | Fiber: 2g | Sugars: 5g | Protein: 6g

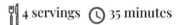

Cauliflower Steak with Walnut Pesto

🍴 4 servings   🕐 35 minutes

INGREDIENTS

- 1 large head cauliflower, sliced into steaks
- 1/2 cup walnuts
- 1/4 cup fresh basil leaves
- 2 cloves garlic
- 1/4 cup grated Parmesan cheese
- 1/4 cup olive oil
- Salt and pepper to taste
- Lemon wedges for serving

DIRECTIONS

1. Preheat the oven to 400°F (200°C).
2. In a food processor, blend walnuts, basil, garlic, Parmesan, and olive oil until smooth. Season with salt and pepper.
3. Place cauliflower steaks on a baking sheet. Brush with walnut pesto.
4. Bake for 20 minutes or until cauliflower is tender and golden.
5. Serve with lemon wedges.

Nutritional Information per serving: Calories: 250 | Total Fat: 22g | Saturated Fat: 4g | Trans Fat: 0g | Polyunsaturated Fat: 8g | Monounsaturated Fat: 9g | Cholesterol: 5mg | Sodium: 180mg | Carbohydrates: 9g | Fiber: 3g | Sugars: 3g | Protein: 7g

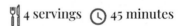

Roasted Vegetable and Quinoa Bowl

🍴 4 servings   🕐 45 minutes

INGREDIENTS

- 1 cup quinoa, cooked
- 1 red bell pepper, chopped
- 1 zucchini, chopped
- 1 yellow squash, chopped
- 1 red onion, chopped
- 2 tablespoons olive oil
- 1 teaspoon smoked paprika
- Salt and pepper to taste
- Fresh parsley for garnish

DIRECTIONS

1. Preheat oven to 400°F (200°C).
2. Toss bell pepper, zucchini, squash, and onion with olive oil, smoked paprika, salt, and pepper.
3. Spread vegetables on a baking sheet and roast for 30 minutes, stirring halfway through.
4. Serve roasted vegetables over cooked quinoa.

5. Garnish with fresh parsley.

Nutritional Information per serving: Calories: 240 | Total Fat: 8g | Saturated Fat: 1g | Trans Fat: 0g | Polyunsaturated Fat: 1g | Monounsaturated Fat: 5g | Cholesterol: 0mg | Sodium: 80mg | Carbohydrates: 36g | Fiber: 5g | Sugars: 5g | Protein: 8g

Ginger Soy Glazed Salmon

🍴 4 servings   🕐 35 minutes

INGREDIENTS

- 4 salmon fillets
- 2 tablespoons soy sauce (low sodium)
- 1 tablespoon honey
- 1 tablespoon fresh ginger, grated
- 2 cloves garlic, minced
- 1 teaspoon sesame oil
- 1 tablespoon olive oil
- Sesame seeds for garnish
- Green onions, sliced for garnish

DIRECTIONS

1. Preheat the oven to 375°F (190°C).
2. In a bowl, whisk together soy sauce, honey, ginger, garlic, and sesame oil.
3. Place salmon fillets in a baking dish. Pour the marinade over the salmon.
4. Let marinate for 10 minutes.
5. Drizzle olive oil over the salmon.
6. Bake for 15-20 minutes, or until salmon is cooked through and flakes easily.
7. Garnish with sesame seeds and green onions.
8. Serve with steamed vegetables or brown rice.

Nutritional Information per serving: Calories: 280 | Total Fat: 13g | Saturated Fat: 2g | Trans Fat: 0g | Polyunsaturated Fat: 5g | Monounsaturated Fat: 5g | Cholesterol: 70mg | Sodium: 320mg | Carbohydrates: 7g | Fiber: 0.5g | Sugars: 5g | Protein: 34g

Hearty Vegetable and Lentil Stew

🍴 6 servings   🕐 55 minutes

INGREDIENTS

- 1 cup brown lentils, rinsed
- 1 onion, chopped
- 2 carrots, diced
- 2 celery stalks, diced
- 1 bell pepper, chopped
- 3 cloves garlic, minced

- 1 can diced tomatoes
- 6 cups vegetable broth
- 2 teaspoons thyme
- 2 tablespoons olive oil
- Salt and pepper to taste
- Fresh parsley, chopped for garnish

DIRECTIONS

1. Heat olive oil in a large pot over medium heat.
2. Sauté onion, carrots, celery, bell pepper, and garlic until softened.
3. Add lentils, diced tomatoes, thyme, and vegetable broth.
4. Bring to a boil, then reduce heat and simmer for 30-40 minutes, until lentils are tender.
5. Season with salt and pepper.
6. Garnish with fresh parsley before serving.

Nutritional Information per serving: Calories: 220 | Total Fat: 5g | Saturated Fat: 0.7g | Trans Fat: 0g | Polyunsaturated Fat: 0.7g | Monounsaturated Fat: 3.3g | Cholesterol: 0mg | Sodium: 480mg | Carbohydrates: 33g | Fiber: 13g | Sugars: 6g | Protein: 11g

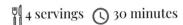

Asian-Style Grilled Tofu with Greens

🍴 4 servings 🕐 30 minutes

INGREDIENTS

- 14 oz firm tofu, pressed and sliced
- 2 tablespoons soy sauce (low sodium)
- 1 tablespoon honey or maple syrup
- 1 tablespoon fresh ginger, grated
- 2 cloves garlic, minced
- 1 teaspoon sesame oil
- 4 cups mixed greens (such as bok choy, spinach, and kale)
- 1 tablespoon olive oil
- Sesame seeds for garnish

DIRECTIONS

1. In a bowl, whisk together soy sauce, honey or maple syrup, ginger, garlic, and sesame oil.
2. Marinate tofu slices in the mixture for at least 15 minutes.
3. Preheat a grill or grill pan over medium heat. Grill tofu for about 5 minutes on each side, or until golden and crispy.
4. Meanwhile, heat olive oil in a large skillet. Sauté mixed greens until wilted.
5. Serve grilled tofu on top of the greens. Sprinkle with sesame seeds.

Nutritional Information per serving: Calories: 200 | Total Fat: 10g | Saturated Fat: 1.5g | Trans Fat: 0g | Polyunsaturated Fat: 4g |

Monounsaturated Fat: 4g | Cholesterol: 0mg | Sodium: 320mg | Carbohydrates: 15g | Fiber: 3g | Sugars: 6g | Protein: 14g

Moroccan Vegetable Tagine

🍴 6 servings 🕐 55 minutes

INGREDIENTS

- 2 carrots, chopped
- 2 zucchini, chopped
- 1 eggplant, chopped
- 1 onion, chopped
- 2 cloves garlic, minced
- 1 can chickpeas, drained and rinsed
- 1 can diced tomatoes
- 4 cups vegetable broth
- 2 teaspoons cumin
- 1 teaspoon paprika
- 1 teaspoon cinnamon
- 1/2 teaspoon ginger
- 2 tablespoons olive oil
- Salt and pepper to taste
- Fresh cilantro for garnish

DIRECTIONS

1. Heat olive oil in a large pot or tagine over medium heat. Sauté onion and garlic until translucent.
2. Add carrots, zucchini, and eggplant. Cook for 5 minutes.
3. Stir in chickpeas, diced tomatoes, vegetable broth, cumin, paprika, cinnamon, and ginger.
4. Bring to a simmer, cover, and cook for 30 minutes, or until vegetables are tender.
5. Season with salt and pepper.
6. Garnish with fresh cilantro before serving.

Nutritional Information per serving: Calories: 210 | Total Fat: 5g | Saturated Fat: 0.7g | Trans Fat: 0g | Polyunsaturated Fat: 1g | Monounsaturated Fat: 3g | Cholesterol: 0mg | Sodium: 480mg | Carbohydrates: 35g | Fiber: 10g | Sugars: 10g | Protein: 9g

Miso-Glazed Cod with Bok Choy

🍴 4 servings 🕐 30 minutes

INGREDIENTS

- 4 cod fillets (about 6 ounces each)
- 3 tablespoons white miso paste
- 1 tablespoon honey or maple syrup
- 1 tablespoon rice vinegar

- 1 tablespoon soy sauce (low sodium)
- 1 teaspoon sesame oil
- 2 cloves garlic, minced
- 1 teaspoon fresh ginger, grated
- 2 bunches bok choy, trimmed and halved lengthwise
- 1 tablespoon olive oil
- Sesame seeds for garnish
- Sliced green onions for garnish

DIRECTIONS

1. Preheat your oven to 400°F (200°C).
2. In a small bowl, whisk together miso paste, honey or maple syrup, rice vinegar, soy sauce, sesame oil, garlic, and ginger to make the glaze.
3. Place cod fillets on a baking sheet lined with parchment paper. Brush the fillets generously with the miso glaze.
4. Bake in the preheated oven for about 12-15 minutes, or until the cod is flaky and cooked through.
5. While the fish is baking, heat olive oil in a large skillet over medium heat. Add bok choy and sauté for 3-5 minutes on each side, or until tender and lightly browned.
6. Serve the miso-glazed cod with the sautéed bok choy, garnished with sesame seeds and green onions.

Nutritional Information per serving: Calories: 280 | Total Fat: 9g | Saturated Fat: 1.5g | Trans Fat: 0g | Polyunsaturated Fat: 3g | Monounsaturated Fat: 4g | Cholesterol: 65mg | Sodium: 700mg | Carbohydrates: 14g | Fiber: 2g | Sugars: 7g | Protein: 36g

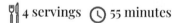

Spaghetti Squash with Spinach and Feta

🍴 4 servings 🕐 55 minutes

INGREDIENTS

- 1 large spaghetti squash
- 4 cups fresh spinach
- 1/2 cup crumbled feta cheese
- 2 cloves garlic, minced
- 2 tablespoons olive oil
- Salt and pepper to taste
- Red pepper flakes (optional)
- Grated Parmesan cheese for garnish (optional)

DIRECTIONS

1. Preheat the oven to 400°F (200°C). Halve the spaghetti squash lengthwise and scoop out the seeds.
2. Place the squash halves cut-side down on a baking sheet. Roast for 35-40 minutes, or until the flesh is tender and easily shreds with a fork.

3. While the squash is roasting, heat olive oil in a skillet over medium heat. Add garlic and sauté for 1 minute.
4. Add spinach to the skillet and sauté until wilted. Season with salt, pepper, and red pepper flakes if using.
5. Once the squash is done, use a fork to scrape the inside to create spaghetti-like strands.
6. Mix the squash strands with the sautéed spinach and feta cheese.
7. Serve warm, garnished with grated Parmesan cheese if desired.

Nutritional Information per serving: Calories: 180 | Total Fat: 10g | Saturated Fat: 3g | Trans Fat: 0g | Polyunsaturated Fat: 1g | Monounsaturated Fat: 5g | Cholesterol: 15mg | Sodium: 300mg | Carbohydrates: 20g | Fiber: 4g | Sugars: 8g | Protein: 6g

Quinoa-Stuffed Bell Peppers

🍴 4 servings 🕐 45 minutes

INGREDIENTS

- 1 cup quinoa, rinsed and drained
- 4 large bell peppers, halved and seeds removed
- 1 can (15 oz) black beans, drained and rinsed
- 1 cup corn kernels (fresh or frozen)
- 1 cup diced tomatoes
- 1 cup diced zucchini
- 1/2 cup diced red onion
- 2 cloves garlic, minced
- 1 teaspoon ground cumin
- 1 teaspoon chili powder
- 1/2 teaspoon smoked paprika
- Salt and pepper to taste
- 1 cup shredded low-fat cheddar cheese (optional)
- Fresh cilantro, chopped, for garnish

DIRECTIONS

1. Preheat the oven to 375°F (190°C).
2. In a saucepan, combine quinoa with 2 cups of water. Bring to a boil, then reduce heat, cover, and simmer for 15 minutes or until quinoa is cooked and water is absorbed.
3. While quinoa is cooking, prepare the bell peppers by cutting them in half and removing seeds.
4. In a large mixing bowl, combine cooked quinoa, black beans, corn, diced tomatoes, zucchini, red onion, minced garlic, cumin, chili powder, smoked paprika, salt, and pepper. Mix well.
5. Stuff each bell pepper half with the quinoa mixture.
6. Place stuffed bell peppers in a baking dish. If desired, sprinkle shredded cheddar cheese on top.

7. Bake in the preheated oven for 25 minutes or until the peppers are tender.
8. Garnish with fresh chopped cilantro before serving.

Nutritional Information per serving: Calories: 320 | Total Fat: 5g | Saturated Fat: 2g | Trans Fat: 0g | Polyunsaturated Fat: 1g | Monounsaturated Fat: 1g | Cholesterol: 10mg | Sodium: 350mg | Carbohydrates: 60g | Fiber: 12g | Sugars: 7g | Protein: 13g

Lemon Garlic Shrimp with Quinoa

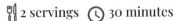 2 servings   🕐 30 minutes

INGREDIENTS

- 1 cup quinoa, rinsed and drained
- 1 pound large shrimp, peeled and deveined
- 3 tablespoons olive oil
- 4 cloves garlic, minced
- Zest of 1 lemon
- Juice of 1 lemon
- 1 teaspoon dried oregano
- 1/2 teaspoon red pepper flakes (optional)
- Salt and black pepper to taste
- 2 cups baby spinach
- 1 cup cherry tomatoes, halved
- Fresh parsley, chopped, for garnish

DIRECTIONS

1. Cook quinoa according to package instructions.
2. In a large skillet, heat olive oil over medium-high heat. Add minced garlic and cook for 1-2 minutes until fragrant.
3. Add shrimp to the skillet, stirring occasionally, until they turn pink and opaque, about 3-4 minutes.
4. Stir in lemon zest, lemon juice, dried oregano, red pepper flakes (if using), salt, and black pepper.
5. Add baby spinach and cherry tomatoes to the skillet. Cook for an additional 2-3 minutes until the spinach wilts and tomatoes soften.
6. Serve the lemon garlic shrimp over a bed of cooked quinoa.
7. Garnish with fresh chopped parsley.

Nutritional Information per serving: Calories: 450 | Total Fat: 15g | Saturated Fat: 2g | Trans Fat: 0g | Polyunsaturated Fat: 2g | Monounsaturated Fat: 9g | Cholesterol: 250mg | Sodium: 350mg | Carbohydrates: 45g | Fiber: 7g | Sugars: 2g | Protein: 35g

CHAPTER 5: SALADS

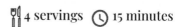
Kale and Avocado Salad with Lemon Tahini Dressing

🍴 4 servings   🕐 15 minutes

INGREDIENTS
- 4 cups kale, chopped
- 1 ripe avocado, diced
- 1/2 red onion, thinly sliced
- 1/4 cup sunflower seeds
- For the Dressing:
- 3 tablespoons tahini
- Juice of 1 lemon
- 1 clove garlic, minced
- 2 tablespoons water
- Salt and pepper to taste

DIRECTIONS
1. In a large bowl, combine the chopped kale, diced avocado, and red onion.
2. In a small bowl, whisk together tahini, lemon juice, minced garlic, and water to create a smooth dressing. Season with salt and pepper.
3. Pour the dressing over the salad and toss to coat evenly.
4. Sprinkle sunflower seeds on top of the salad before serving.

Nutritional Information per serving: Calories: 220 | Total Fat: 17g | Saturated Fat: 2.5g | Trans Fat: 0g | Polyunsaturated Fat: 4g | Monounsaturated Fat: 10g | Cholesterol: 0mg | Sodium: 60mg | Carbohydrates: 15g | Fiber: 6g | Sugars: 2g | Protein: 6g

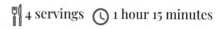
Roasted Beet and Orange Salad with Walnuts

🍴 4 servings   🕐 1 hour 15 minutes

INGREDIENTS
- 4 medium beets, roasted and sliced
- 2 oranges, peeled and segments
- 1/4 cup walnuts, toasted and chopped
- 4 cups mixed salad greens
- For the Dressing:
- 3 tablespoons olive oil
- 1 tablespoon balsamic vinegar
- 1 teaspoon honey
- Salt and pepper to taste

DIRECTIONS
1. To roast the beets, wrap each beet in aluminum foil and bake in a preheated 400°F (200°C) oven for about 1 hour or until tender. Once cooled, peel and slice.
2. Arrange mixed salad greens on a serving platter or in a large bowl.
3. Top with roasted beet slices and orange segments.
4. In a small bowl, whisk together olive oil, balsamic vinegar, honey, salt, and pepper to make the dressing.
5. Drizzle the dressing over the salad and sprinkle with toasted walnuts.

Nutritional Information per serving: Calories: 210 | Total Fat: 14g | Saturated Fat: 1.5g | Trans Fat: 0g | Polyunsaturated Fat: 5g | Monounsaturated Fat: 7g | Cholesterol: 0mg | Sodium: 85mg | Carbohydrates: 20g | Fiber: 5g | Sugars: 13g | Protein: 4g

Quinoa Tabbouleh Salad

🍴 4 servings   🕐 35 minutes

INGREDIENTS
- 1 cup quinoa, cooked and cooled
- 1 cucumber, diced
- 2 tomatoes, diced
- 1/2 cup fresh parsley, chopped
- 1/4 cup fresh mint, chopped
- 1/4 cup lemon juice
- 1/4 cup olive oil
- 2 cloves garlic, minced
- Salt and pepper to taste

DIRECTIONS
1. In a large bowl, combine cooked quinoa, diced cucumber, diced tomatoes, chopped parsley, and chopped mint.
2. In a small bowl, whisk together lemon juice, olive oil, minced garlic, salt, and pepper to make the dressing.
3. Pour the dressing over the quinoa mixture and toss to combine.
4. Chill in the refrigerator for at least 30 minutes before serving to allow flavors to meld.

Nutritional Information per serving: Calories: 280 | Total Fat: 15g | Saturated Fat: 2g | Trans Fat: 0g | Polyunsaturated Fat: 2g | Monounsaturated Fat: 10g | Cholesterol: 0mg | Sodium: 15mg | Carbohydrates: 33g | Fiber: 5g | Sugars: 3g | Protein: 6g

Arugula, Pear, and Blue Cheese Salad

🍴 4 servings 🕐 15 minutes

INGREDIENTS

- 4 cups arugula
- 2 ripe pears, sliced
- 1/2 cup blue cheese, crumbled
- 1/4 cup walnuts, toasted and chopped
- For the Dressing:
- 3 tablespoons olive oil
- 1 tablespoon apple cider vinegar
- 1 teaspoon Dijon mustard
- 1 teaspoon honey
- Salt and pepper to taste

DIRECTIONS

1. In a large bowl, combine arugula, sliced pears, crumbled blue cheese, and toasted walnuts.
2. In a small bowl, whisk together olive oil, apple cider vinegar, Dijon mustard, honey, salt, and pepper to create the dressing.
3. Drizzle the dressing over the salad and toss gently to combine.
4. Serve immediately.

Nutritional Information per serving: Calories: 240 | Total Fat: 18g | Saturated Fat: 4g | Trans Fat: 0g | Polyunsaturated Fat: 4g | Monounsaturated Fat: 9g | Cholesterol: 10mg | Sodium: 280mg | Carbohydrates: 16g | Fiber: 3g | Sugars: 10g | Protein: 6g

Grilled Peach and Spinach Salad

🍴 4 servings 🕐 25 minutes

INGREDIENTS

- 4 peaches, halved and pitted
- 6 cups baby spinach
- 1/4 cup goat cheese, crumbled
- 1/4 cup almonds, sliced and toasted
- For the Dressing:
- 3 tablespoons olive oil
- 1 tablespoon balsamic vinegar
- 1 teaspoon honey
- Salt and pepper to taste

DIRECTIONS

1. Preheat grill to medium heat. Grill peach halves for about 4-5 minutes per side, or until they have grill marks and are slightly softened.

2. In a large bowl, combine baby spinach, grilled peaches (sliced), crumbled goat cheese, and toasted almonds.
3. In a small bowl, whisk together olive oil, balsamic vinegar, honey, salt, and pepper to make the dressing.
4. Drizzle the dressing over the salad and toss gently to combine.
5. Serve immediately.

Nutritional Information per serving: Calories: 180 | Total Fat: 7g | Saturated Fat: 1g | Trans Fat: 0g | Polyunsaturated Fat: 3g | Monounsaturated Fat: 2g | Cholesterol: 3mg | Sodium: 40mg | Carbohydrates: 27g | Fiber: 5g | Sugars: 18g | Protein: 6g

Cucumber and Dill Salad with Yogurt Dressing

🍴 4 servings 🕐 10 minutes

INGREDIENTS

- 2 large cucumbers, thinly sliced
- 1/4 cup fresh dill, chopped
- 1/4 cup red onion, thinly sliced
- For the Dressing:
- 1/2 cup plain Greek yogurt
- 2 tablespoons lemon juice
- 1 clove garlic, minced
- Salt and pepper to taste

DIRECTIONS

1. In a large bowl, combine sliced cucumbers, chopped dill, and sliced red onion.
2. In a small bowl, whisk together Greek yogurt, lemon juice, minced garlic, salt, and pepper to make the dressing.
3. Pour the dressing over the cucumber mixture and toss gently to combine.
4. Chill in the refrigerator for at least 1 hour before serving to allow flavors to meld.

Nutritional Information per serving: Calories: 70 | Total Fat: 1g | Saturated Fat: 0.5g | Trans Fat: 0g | Polyunsaturated Fat: 0g | Monounsaturated Fat: 0g | Cholesterol: 3mg | Sodium: 25mg | Carbohydrates: 11g | Fiber: 1g | Sugars: 6g | Protein: 4g

Roasted Carrot and Chickpea Salad

🍴 4 servings 🕐 40 minutes

INGREDIENTS

- 4 large carrots, peeled and sliced
- 1 can chickpeas, drained and rinsed
- 2 tablespoons olive oil
- 1 teaspoon cumin
- Salt and pepper to taste
- 4 cups mixed greens
- For the Dressing:
- 3 tablespoons olive oil
- 2 tablespoons lemon juice
- 1 teaspoon honey
- 1 clove garlic, minced
- Salt and pepper to taste

DIRECTIONS

1. Preheat the oven to 400°F (200°C).
2. Toss carrots and chickpeas with olive oil, cumin, salt, and pepper. Spread on a baking sheet.
3. Roast for 25 minutes, or until carrots are tender and chickpeas are crispy.
4. In a large bowl, mix roasted carrots and chickpeas with mixed greens.
5. In a small bowl, whisk together olive oil, lemon juice, honey, minced garlic, salt, and pepper for the dressing.
6. Drizzle the dressing over the salad and toss to combine.
7. Serve immediately.

Nutritional Information per serving: Calories: 260 | Total Fat: 14g | Saturated Fat: 2g | Trans Fat: 0g | Polyunsaturated Fat: 2g | Monounsaturated Fat: 10g | Cholesterol: 0mg | Sodium: 320mg | Carbohydrates: 30g | Fiber: 8g | Sugars: 10g | Protein: 7g

Watermelon and Feta Salad with Mint

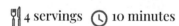

🍴 4 servings 🕐 10 minutes

INGREDIENTS

- 4 cups watermelon, cubed
- 1/2 cup feta cheese, crumbled
- 1/4 cup fresh mint, chopped
- 2 tablespoons olive oil
- 1 tablespoon balsamic vinegar
- Salt and pepper to taste

DIRECTIONS

1. In a large bowl, combine cubed watermelon, crumbled feta cheese, and chopped mint.
2. In a small bowl, whisk together olive oil, balsamic vinegar, salt, and pepper to make the dressing.
3. Drizzle the dressing over the watermelon mixture and toss gently to combine.
4. Serve chilled for a refreshing salad.

Nutritional Information per serving: Calories: 160 | Total Fat: 10g | Saturated Fat: 3g | Trans Fat: 0g | Polyunsaturated Fat: 1g | Monounsaturated Fat: 6g | Cholesterol: 15mg | Sodium: 170mg | Carbohydrates: 16g | Fiber: 1g | Sugars: 13g | Protein: 4g

Asian Cabbage Slaw with Peanut Dressing

🍴 4 servings 🕐 15 minutes

INGREDIENTS

- 4 cups cabbage, shredded (mix of red and green)
- 1 carrot, julienned
- 1 red bell pepper, thinly sliced
- 1/4 cup green onions, chopped
- 1/4 cup cilantro, chopped
- For the Dressing:
- 3 tablespoons peanut butter
- 2 tablespoons soy sauce (low sodium)
- 1 tablespoon rice vinegar
- 1 tablespoon honey or maple syrup
- 1 clove garlic, minced
- 1 teaspoon fresh ginger, grated
- Water to thin, if needed

DIRECTIONS

1. In a large bowl, combine shredded cabbage, julienned carrot, sliced red bell pepper, chopped green onions, and cilantro.
2. In a small bowl, whisk together peanut butter, soy sauce, rice vinegar, honey or maple syrup, minced garlic, and grated ginger to make the dressing. Add a little water if needed to reach a pourable consistency.
3. Pour the dressing over the slaw and toss well to coat.
4. Chill in the refrigerator for about 30 minutes before serving to allow flavors to meld.

Nutritional Information per serving: Calories: 180 | Total Fat: 8g | Saturated Fat: 1.5g | Trans Fat: 0g | Polyunsaturated Fat: 2.5g | Monounsaturated Fat: 4g | Cholesterol: 0mg | Sodium: 430mg | Carbohydrates: 24g | Fiber: 4g | Sugars: 14g | Protein: 6g

Brussels Sprout and Cranberry Salad

🍴 4 servings 🕐 20 minutes

INGREDIENTS

- 4 cups Brussels sprouts, trimmed and thinly sliced
- 1/2 cup dried cranberries

- 1/4 cup walnuts, chopped and toasted
- 1/4 cup Parmesan cheese, shaved
- For the Dressing:
- 3 tablespoons olive oil
- 2 tablespoons apple cider vinegar
- 1 tablespoon honey
- 1 teaspoon Dijon mustard
- Salt and pepper to taste

DIRECTIONS

1. In a large bowl, combine thinly sliced Brussels sprouts, dried cranberries, toasted walnuts, and shaved Parmesan cheese.
2. In a small bowl, whisk together olive oil, apple cider vinegar, honey, Dijon mustard, salt, and pepper to create the dressing.
3. Drizzle the dressing over the salad and toss to coat evenly.
4. Let the salad sit for about 10 minutes before serving to allow flavors to meld.

Nutritional Information per serving: Calories: 230 | Total Fat: 15g | Saturated Fat: 3g | Trans Fat: 0g | Polyunsaturated Fat: 3g | Monounsaturated Fat: 8g | Cholesterol: 5mg | Sodium: 150mg | Carbohydrates: 22g | Fiber: 4g | Sugars: 14g | Protein: 6g

Barley Salad with Roasted Vegetables and Lemon Vinaigrette

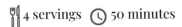

🍴 4 servings 🕐 50 minutes

INGREDIENTS

- 1 cup barley, cooked and cooled
- 2 carrots, diced
- 1 zucchini, diced
- 1 red bell pepper, diced
- 2 tablespoons olive oil
- For the Lemon Vinaigrette:
- 3 tablespoons olive oil
- Juice of 1 lemon
- 1 garlic clove, minced
- 1 teaspoon honey
- Salt and pepper to taste

DIRECTIONS

1. Preheat the oven to 400°F (200°C).
2. Toss diced carrots, zucchini, and red bell pepper with 2 tablespoons olive oil. Spread on a baking sheet and roast for 30 minutes, or until vegetables are tender.
3. In a large bowl, mix cooked barley with roasted vegetables.
4. In a small bowl, whisk together olive oil, lemon juice, minced garlic, honey, salt, and pepper to make the vinaigrette.
5. Drizzle the vinaigrette over the barley and vegetable mixture. Toss to combine.

6. Serve the salad warm or at room temperature.

Nutritional Information per serving: Calories: 280 | Total Fat: 14g | Saturated Fat: 2g | Trans Fat: 0g | Polyunsaturated Fat: 2g | Monounsaturated Fat: 10g | Cholesterol: 0mg | Sodium: 50mg | Carbohydrates: 36g | Fiber: 8g | Sugars: 6g | Protein: 6g

Mediterranean Quinoa and White Bean Salad

🍴 4 servings 🕐 15 minutes

INGREDIENTS

- 1 cup quinoa, cooked and cooled
- 1 can white beans, drained and rinsed
- 1 cucumber, diced
- 1/2 cup cherry tomatoes, halved
- 1/4 cup Kalamata olives, sliced
- 1/4 cup red onion, finely chopped
- 1/4 cup feta cheese, crumbled
- For the Dressing:
- 3 tablespoons olive oil
- 2 tablespoons red wine vinegar
- 1 teaspoon dried oregano
- Salt and pepper to taste

DIRECTIONS

1. In a large bowl, combine cooked quinoa, white beans, diced cucumber, halved cherry tomatoes, sliced olives, chopped red onion, and crumbled feta cheese.
2. In a small bowl, whisk together olive oil, red wine vinegar, dried oregano, salt, and pepper to make the dressing.
3. Pour the dressing over the salad and toss to combine.
4. Chill in the refrigerator for about 30 minutes before serving to allow flavors to meld.

Nutritional Information per serving: Calories: 330 | Total Fat: 14g | Saturated Fat: 3g | Trans Fat: 0g | Polyunsaturated Fat: 2g | Monounsaturated Fat: 9g | Cholesterol: 10mg | Sodium: 320mg | Carbohydrates: 42g | Fiber: 8g | Sugars: 3g | Protein: 13g

Endive and Roasted Pepper Salad with Goat Cheese

🍴 4 servings 🕐 15 minutes

INGREDIENTS

- 4 endives, leaves separated
- 1 jar roasted red peppers, drained and sliced
- 1/4 cup goat cheese, crumbled

- 1/4 cup walnuts, toasted and chopped
- For the Dressing:
- 3 tablespoons olive oil
- 1 tablespoon balsamic vinegar
- 1 teaspoon honey
- Salt and pepper to taste

DIRECTIONS

1. Arrange endive leaves on a serving platter.
2. Top with sliced roasted red peppers, crumbled goat cheese, and toasted walnuts.
3. In a small bowl, whisk together olive oil, balsamic vinegar, honey, salt, and pepper to make the dressing.
4. Drizzle the dressing over the salad just before serving.

Nutritional Information per serving: Calories: 210 Total Fat: 17g | Saturated Fat: 4g | Trans Fat: 0g Polyunsaturated Fat: 3g | Monounsaturated Fat: 9g Cholesterol: 10mg | Sodium: 300mg | Carbohydrates: 10g | Fiber: 4g | Sugars: 5g | Protein: 6g

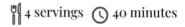

Rainbow Chard and Roasted Sweet Potato Salad with Pomegranate Seeds

🍴 4 servings 🕐 40 minutes

INGREDIENTS

- 2 sweet potatoes, peeled and cubed
- 1 bunch rainbow chard, chopped
- 1/4 cup pomegranate seeds
- 1/4 cup almonds, sliced and toasted
- For the Dressing:
- 3 tablespoons olive oil
- 2 tablespoons apple cider vinegar
- 1 tablespoon maple syrup
- 1 teaspoon Dijon mustard
- Salt and pepper to taste

DIRECTIONS

1. Preheat the oven to 400°F (200°C).
2. Toss cubed sweet potatoes with 1 tablespoon olive oil, salt, and pepper. Spread on a baking sheet and roast for 25 minutes, or until tender.
3. In a large bowl, combine chopped rainbow chard, roasted sweet potatoes, pomegranate seeds, and toasted almonds.
4. In a small bowl, whisk together olive oil, apple cider vinegar, maple syrup, Dijon mustard, salt, and pepper to make the dressing.
5. Drizzle the dressing over the salad and toss gently to combine.
6. Serve immediately.

Nutritional Information per serving: Calories: 250 Total Fat: 14g | Saturated Fat: 2g | Trans Fat: 0g Polyunsaturated Fat: 2g | Monounsaturated Fat: 10g Cholesterol: 0mg | Sodium: 75mg | Carbohydrates: 29g | Fiber: 5g | Sugars: 12g | Protein: 5g

Spinach and Strawberry Salad with Balsamic Vinaigrette

🍴 4 servings 🕐 15 minutes

INGREDIENTS

- 8 cups baby spinach, washed and dried
- 1 pint strawberries, hulled and sliced
- 1/2 cup sliced almonds, toasted
- 1/4 cup crumbled feta cheese (optional)
- Balsamic Vinaigrette:
- 3 tablespoons balsamic vinegar
- 2 tablespoons extra-virgin olive oil
- 1 teaspoon Dijon mustard
- 1 teaspoon honey
- Salt and black pepper to taste

DIRECTIONS

1. In a large salad bowl, combine baby spinach, sliced strawberries, toasted sliced almonds, and crumbled feta cheese (if using).
2.
3. In a small bowl, whisk together balsamic vinegar, olive oil, Dijon mustard, honey, salt, and black pepper to make the vinaigrette.
4. Drizzle the balsamic vinaigrette over the salad and toss gently to coat.
5. Serve immediately as a refreshing and heart-healthy salad.

Nutritional Information per serving: Calories: 180 Total Fat: 12g | Saturated Fat: 1.5g | Trans Fat: 0g Polyunsaturated Fat: 2.5g | Monounsaturated Fat: 7g Cholesterol: 0mg | Sodium: 70mg | Carbohydrates: 16g | Fiber: 5g | Sugars: 8g | Protein: 5g

Mediterranean Chickpea Salad

🍴 4 servings 🕐 15 minutes

INGREDIENTS

- 1 can (15 oz) chickpeas, drained and rinsed
- 1 cup cherry tomatoes, halved
- 1 cucumber, diced
- 1/2 red onion, finely chopped
- 1/2 cup Kalamata olives, pitted and sliced
- 1/2 cup crumbled feta cheese

- Fresh parsley, chopped, for garnish
- Lemon Vinaigrette:
- 3 tablespoons extra-virgin olive oil
- Juice of 1 lemon
- 1 teaspoon dried oregano
- Salt and black pepper to taste

DIRECTIONS

1. In a large bowl, combine chickpeas, cherry tomatoes, cucumber, red onion, Kalamata olives, and crumbled feta cheese.
2. In a small bowl, whisk together olive oil, lemon juice, dried oregano, salt, and black pepper to make the lemon vinaigrette.
3. Drizzle the lemon vinaigrette over the salad and toss gently to combine.
4. Garnish with fresh chopped parsley before serving.
5. Enjoy this Mediterranean-inspired chickpea salad for a light and heart-healthy meal.

Nutritional Information per serving: Calories: 280 | Total Fat: 18g | Saturated Fat: 4g | Trans Fat: 0g | Polyunsaturated Fat: 2.5g | Monounsaturated Fat: 11g | Cholesterol: 15mg | Sodium: 480mg | Carbohydrates: 26g | Fiber: 7g | Sugars: 6g | Protein: 8g

CHAPTER 6: MEAT AND POULTRY

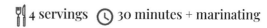

Grilled Lemon-Herb Chicken Skewers

🍴 4 servings 🕐 30 minutes + marinating

INGREDIENTS
- 4 boneless, skinless chicken breasts, cut into cubes
- 2 lemons, juice and zest
- 2 tablespoons olive oil
- 2 cloves garlic, minced
- 1 tablespoon fresh rosemary, chopped
- 1 tablespoon fresh thyme, chopped
- Salt and pepper to taste
- Wooden skewers, soaked in water

DIRECTIONS
1. In a bowl, combine lemon juice and zest, olive oil, garlic, rosemary, thyme, salt, and pepper.
2. Add chicken cubes to the marinade and refrigerate for at least 30 minutes, or up to 4 hours.
3. Preheat grill to medium-high heat.
4. Thread marinated chicken onto skewers.
5. Grill skewers for 10 minutes, turning occasionally, until chicken is cooked through and has grill marks.
6. Serve hot.

Nutritional Information per serving: Calories: 220 | Total Fat: 9g | Saturated Fat: 1.5g | Trans Fat: 0g | Polyunsaturated Fat: 1g | Monounsaturated Fat: 6g | Cholesterol: 80mg | Sodium: 150mg | Carbohydrates: 3g | Fiber: 1g | Sugars: 1g | Protein: 31g

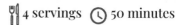

Turkey and Spinach Meatballs in Marinara Sauce

🍴 4 servings 🕐 50 minutes

INGREDIENTS
- 1 lb ground turkey
- 2 cups fresh spinach, finely chopped
- 1 egg
- 1/4 cup whole wheat breadcrumbs
- 2 cloves garlic, minced
- 1 teaspoon Italian seasoning
- Salt and pepper to taste
- 2 cups marinara sauce, low-sodium
- Fresh basil for garnish

DIRECTIONS
1. Preheat the oven to 375°F (190°C).
2. In a bowl, mix together ground turkey, spinach, egg, breadcrumbs, garlic, Italian seasoning, salt, and pepper.
3. Form mixture into meatballs and place on a baking sheet lined with parchment paper.
4. Bake for 20 minutes.
5. Heat marinara sauce in a saucepan. Add cooked meatballs to the sauce and simmer for 10 minutes.
6. Garnish with fresh basil before serving.

Nutritional Information per serving: Calories: 230 | Total Fat: 9g | Saturated Fat: 2g | Trans Fat: 0g | Polyunsaturated Fat: 2g | Monounsaturated Fat: 4g | Cholesterol: 100mg | Sodium: 470mg | Carbohydrates: 14g | Fiber: 3g | Sugars: 6g | Protein: 26g

Stuffed Chicken Breast with Spinach and Ricotta

🍴 4 servings 🕐 45 minutes

INGREDIENTS
- 4 chicken breasts
- 1 cup ricotta cheese
- 2 cups fresh spinach, chopped
- 2 cloves garlic, minced
- 1 teaspoon Italian seasoning
- Salt and pepper to taste
- 2 tablespoons olive oil

DIRECTIONS
1. Preheat the oven to 375°F (190°C).
2. In a bowl, combine ricotta, spinach, garlic, Italian seasoning, salt, and pepper.
3. Cut a pocket into each chicken breast and stuff with the ricotta mixture.
4. Season chicken with salt and pepper.
5. Heat olive oil in a skillet over medium heat. Sear chicken breasts for 3 minutes on each side.
6. Transfer to the oven and bake for 20 minutes, or until chicken is cooked through.
7. Serve hot.

Nutritional Information per serving: Calories: 340 | Total Fat: 15g | Saturated Fat: 4.5g | Trans Fat: 0g | Polyunsaturated Fat: 2g | Monounsaturated Fat: 8g | Cholesterol: 110mg | Sodium: 250mg | Carbohydrates: 4g | Fiber: 1g | Sugars: 1g | Protein: 46g

Turkey Stuffed Bell Peppers

🍴 4 servings   🕐 50 minutes

INGREDIENTS
- 4 bell peppers, tops removed and seeded
- 1 lb ground turkey
- 1 onion, diced
- 2 cloves garlic, minced
- 1 cup cooked brown rice
- 1 can diced tomatoes, drained
- 1 teaspoon cumin
- 1 teaspoon paprika
- Salt and pepper to taste
- 1/2 cup shredded low-fat cheese
- Fresh parsley for garnish

DIRECTIONS
1. Preheat the oven to 375°F (190°C).
2. In a skillet, cook ground turkey, onion, and garlic over medium heat until turkey is browned.
3. Stir in cooked brown rice, chopped tomatoes, cumin, paprika, salt, and pepper.
4. Fill each bell pepper with the turkey mixture. Place in a baking dish.
5. Bake for 25 minutes.
6. Top each pepper with shredded cheese and bake for an additional 5 minutes.
7. Garnish with fresh parsley before serving.

Nutritional Information per serving: Calories: 290 | Total Fat: 9g | Saturated Fat: 3g | Trans Fat: 0g | Polyunsaturated Fat: 2g | Monounsaturated Fat: 3g | Cholesterol: 70mg | Sodium: 320mg | Carbohydrates: 27g | Fiber: 5g | Sugars: 7g | Protein: 29g

Rosemary Garlic Roasted Chicken

🍴 4 servings   🕐 1 hour 30 minutes

INGREDIENTS
- 1 whole chicken (about 4 lbs)
- 4 cloves garlic, minced
- 2 tablespoons fresh rosemary, chopped
- 1 lemon, halved
- 3 tablespoons olive oil
- Salt and pepper to taste

DIRECTIONS
1. Preheat the oven to 375°F (190°C).
2. Rub the chicken with olive oil, garlic, rosemary, salt, and pepper.

3. Place lemon halves inside the chicken cavity.
4. Roast in the oven for about 1 hour and 20 minutes, or until the internal temperature reaches 165°F (75°C).
5. Let the chicken rest for 10 minutes before carving.
6. Serve hot.

Nutritional Information per serving: Calories: 410 | Total Fat: 24g | Saturated Fat: 6g | Trans Fat: 0g | Polyunsaturated Fat: 5g | Monounsaturated Fat: 12g | Cholesterol: 130mg | Sodium: 150mg | Carbohydrates: 3g | Fiber: 1g | Sugars: 1g | Protein: 44g

Slow-Cooked Beef and Vegetable Stew

🍴 6 servings   🕐 8 hour 20 minutes

INGREDIENTS
- 2 lbs beef stew meat, cut into cubes
- 4 carrots, diced
- 3 potatoes, diced
- 1 onion, diced
- 2 cloves garlic, minced
- 4 cups low-sodium beef broth
- 1 can diced tomatoes
- 1 teaspoon thyme
- 1 teaspoon rosemary
- Salt and pepper to taste
- 2 tablespoons olive oil

DIRECTIONS
1. Heat olive oil in a skillet over medium-high heat. Brown the beef cubes on all sides and transfer to a slow cooker.
2. In the slow cooker, add carrots, potatoes, onion, and garlic.
3. Pour in the beef broth and add the diced tomatoes.
4. Stir in thyme, rosemary, salt, and pepper.
5. Cover and cook on low for 8 hours, or until the beef is tender and the vegetables are cooked through.
6. Adjust seasoning if necessary and serve hot.

Nutritional Information per serving: Calories: 350 | Total Fat: 10g | Saturated Fat: 3g | Trans Fat: 0g | Polyunsaturated Fat: 1g | Monounsaturated Fat: 5g | Cholesterol: 90mg | Sodium: 300mg | Carbohydrates: 30g | Fiber: 4g | Sugars: 5g | Protein: 35g

Honey Mustard Glazed Chicken Thighs

🍴 4 servings   🕐 40 minutes

INGREDIENTS

- 8 chicken thighs, skinless and boneless
- 2 tablespoons honey
- 2 tablespoons Dijon mustard
- 1 tablespoon olive oil
- 1 tablespoon apple cider vinegar
- 2 cloves garlic, minced
- Salt and pepper to taste

DIRECTIONS

1. Preheat the oven to 375°F (190°C).
2. In a bowl, mix together honey, Dijon mustard, olive oil, apple cider vinegar, and minced garlic.
3. Season chicken thighs with salt and pepper, then place them in a baking dish.
4. Pour the honey mustard mixture over the chicken, ensuring each piece is well coated.
5. Bake for 25 minutes, or until the chicken is cooked through and the sauce is bubbly.
6. Serve hot with your choice of side, like steamed vegetables or a salad.

Nutritional Information per serving: Calories: 320 | Total Fat: 15g | Saturated Fat: 3.5g | Trans Fat: 0g | Polyunsaturated Fat: 3g | Monounsaturated Fat: 7g | Cholesterol: 145mg | Sodium: 350mg | Carbohydrates: 12g | Fiber: 0g | Sugars: 11g | Protein: 35g

Grilled Turkey Burgers with Avocado

🍴 4 servings 🕐 30 minutes

INGREDIENTS

- 1 lb ground turkey
- 1 ripe avocado, sliced
- 4 whole wheat burger buns
- 1/4 cup Greek yogurt
- 1 tablespoon lemon juice
- 1 teaspoon garlic powder
- Salt and pepper to taste
- Lettuce and tomato slices for garnish

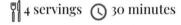

DIRECTIONS

1. In a bowl, mix ground turkey, garlic powder, salt, and pepper. Form into 4 burger patties.
2. Preheat grill to medium-high heat and grill the patties for about 5 minutes on each side or until fully cooked.
3. In a small bowl, mix Greek yogurt and lemon juice to make a creamy sauce.
4. Assemble the burgers on whole wheat buns with turkey patties, sliced avocado, lettuce, tomato, and a dollop of Greek yogurt sauce.
5. Serve immediately.

Nutritional Information per serving: Calories: 320 | Total Fat: 15g | Saturated Fat: 3g | Trans Fat: 0g | Polyunsaturated Fat: 2g | Monounsaturated Fat: 7g | Cholesterol: 80mg | Sodium: 300mg | Carbohydrates: 23g | Fiber: 6g | Sugars: 5g | Protein: 29g

Balsamic Honey Skillet Chicken

🍴 4 servings 🕐 30 minutes

INGREDIENTS

- 4 chicken breasts, boneless and skinless
- 1/4 cup balsamic vinegar
- 2 tablespoons honey
- 1 tablespoon olive oil
- 2 cloves garlic, minced
- 1 teaspoon Italian seasoning
- Salt and pepper to taste

DIRECTIONS

1. In a bowl, whisk together balsamic vinegar, honey, garlic, Italian seasoning, salt, and pepper.
2. Heat olive oil in a skillet over medium heat. Add chicken breasts and cook for 5 minutes on each side, or until browned.
3. Pour the balsamic honey mixture over the chicken in the skillet.
4. Reduce heat to low and simmer for 10 minutes, or until the chicken is cooked through and the sauce has thickened.
5. Serve the chicken drizzled with the sauce from the skillet.

Nutritional Information per serving: Calories: 280 | Total Fat: 7g | Saturated Fat: 1.5g | Trans Fat: 0g | Polyunsaturated Fat: 1g | Monounsaturated Fat: 4g | Cholesterol: 85mg | Sodium: 200mg | Carbohydrates: 15g | Fiber: 0g | Sugars: 13g | Protein: 39g

Asian-Style Turkey Lettuce Wraps

🍴 4 servings 🕐 25 minutes

INGREDIENTS

- 1 lb ground turkey
- 1 tablespoon sesame oil
- 2 cloves garlic, minced
- 1 tablespoon fresh ginger, grated
- 1 red bell pepper, finely diced
- 1/2 cup water chestnuts, diced
- 3 green onions, sliced
- 1/4 cup hoisin sauce
- 2 tablespoons soy sauce (low sodium)

- 1 tablespoon rice vinegar
- 1 head of lettuce, leaves separated (butter lettuce works well)
- Fresh cilantro for garnish

DIRECTIONS

1. Heat sesame oil in a skillet over medium heat. Add garlic and ginger, and sauté for 1 minute.
2. Add ground turkey and cook until browned.
3. Stir in diced bell pepper and water chestnuts, cooking for another 3 minutes.
4. Add hoisin sauce, soy sauce, and rice vinegar. Cook for 2 more minutes, ensuring the mixture is well combined.
5. Spoon the turkey mixture into lettuce leaves. Top with sliced green onions and fresh cilantro.
6. Serve immediately as lettuce wraps.

Nutritional Information per serving: Calories: 220 | Total Fat: 9g | Saturated Fat: 2g | Trans Fat: 0g | Polyunsaturated Fat: 3g | Monounsaturated Fat: 3g | Cholesterol: 60mg | Sodium: 620mg | Carbohydrates: 13g | Fiber: 2g | Sugars: 7g | Protein: 24g

Spiced Chicken and Sweet Potato Bowl

🍴 4 servings 🕐 50 minutes

INGREDIENTS

- 2 large sweet potatoes, peeled and cubed
- 2 chicken breasts, cubed
- 1 tablespoon olive oil
- 1 teaspoon smoked paprika
- 1 teaspoon garlic powder
- 1 teaspoon cumin
- Salt and pepper to taste
- 4 cups mixed greens
- 1 avocado, sliced
- For the Dressing:
- 2 tablespoons Greek yogurt
- 1 tablespoon lime juice
- 1 teaspoon honey
- Salt and pepper to taste

DIRECTIONS

1. Preheat the oven to 400°F (200°C). Toss sweet potatoes with half of the olive oil and a pinch of salt and pepper. Roast for 25-30 minutes until tender.
2. Meanwhile, mix smoked paprika, garlic powder, cumin, salt, and pepper. Coat the chicken cubes with this spice mix.
3. Heat the remaining olive oil in a skillet over medium heat. Add chicken and cook until browned and cooked through.
4. Prepare the dressing by whisking together Greek

yogurt, lime juice, honey, salt, and pepper.
5. Assemble the bowls with a base of mixed greens, roasted sweet potatoes, spiced chicken, and avocado slices.
6. Drizzle with the yogurt dressing before serving.

Nutritional Information per serving: Calories: 350 | Total Fat: 15g | Saturated Fat: 2.5g | Trans Fat: 0g | Polyunsaturated Fat: 2g | Monounsaturated Fat: 9g | Cholesterol: 65mg | Sodium: 200mg | Carbohydrates: 30g | Fiber: 7g | Sugars: 8g | Protein: 27g

Pork Tenderloin with Herbed Quinoa

🍴 4 servings 🕐 45 minutes

INGREDIENTS

- 1 pork tenderloin (about 1 lb)
- 1 tablespoon olive oil
- 1 teaspoon rosemary, chopped
- 1 teaspoon thyme, chopped
- Salt and pepper to taste
- 1 cup quinoa, rinsed
- 2 cups chicken broth, low sodium
- 1/4 cup parsley, chopped

DIRECTIONS

1. Preheat the oven to 375°F (190°C).
2. Season the pork tenderloin with rosemary, thyme, salt, and pepper.
3. Heat olive oil in a skillet over medium-high heat. Sear the pork on all sides.
4. Transfer the pork to the oven and roast for 20 minutes, or until the internal temperature reaches 145°F (63°C).
5. While the pork is roasting, cook quinoa in chicken broth according to package instructions.
6. Stir chopped parsley into the cooked quinoa.
7. Slice the pork and serve it over the herbed quinoa.

Nutritional Information per serving: Calories: 360 | Total Fat: 10g | Saturated Fat: 2g | Trans Fat: 0g | Polyunsaturated Fat: 1.5g | Monounsaturated Fat: 5g | Cholesterol: 75mg | Sodium: 300mg | Carbohydrates: 34g | Fiber: 4g | Sugars: 1g | Protein: 35g

Moroccan Spiced Lamb Chops

🍴 4 servings 🕐 25 minutes + marinating

INGREDIENTS

- 8 lamb chops
- 2 tablespoons olive oil
- 1 teaspoon cumin
- 1 teaspoon coriander
- 1/2 teaspoon cinnamon
- 1/2 teaspoon paprika
- Salt and pepper to taste
- Fresh mint for garnish

DIRECTIONS

1. In a bowl, mix olive oil, cumin, coriander, cinnamon, paprika, salt, and pepper.
2. Coat lamb chops with the spice mixture and let them marinate for at least 30 minutes in the refrigerator.
3. Preheat grill or skillet over medium-high heat.
4. Grill lamb chops for 4-5 minutes on each side, or until they reach your desired level of doneness.
5. Garnish with fresh mint before serving.

Nutritional Information per serving: Calories: 320 | Total Fat: 20g | Saturated Fat: 7g | Trans Fat: 0g | Polyunsaturated Fat: 2g | Monounsaturated Fat: 10g | Cholesterol: 80mg | Sodium: 75mg | Carbohydrates: 1g | Fiber: 0.5g | Sugars: 0.5g | Protein: 35g

Chicken and Black Bean Burrito Bowl

🍴 4 servings   🕐 35 minutes

INGREDIENTS

- 2 chicken breasts, cooked and shredded
- 1 can black beans, drained and rinsed
- 2 cups brown rice, cooked
- 1 avocado, sliced
- 1 cup corn kernels
- 1/2 cup cherry tomatoes, halved
- 1/4 cup red onion, finely chopped
- 1/4 cup fresh cilantro, chopped
- Juice of 1 lime
- Salt and pepper to taste
- 1 teaspoon cumin
- 1/2 teaspoon chili powder
- Greek yogurt for topping (optional)

DIRECTIONS

1. In a bowl, mix shredded chicken with cumin, chili powder, lime juice, salt, and pepper.
2. In serving bowls, evenly distribute cooked brown rice.
3. Top rice with seasoned chicken, black beans, corn, cherry tomatoes, red onion, and avocado slices.
4. Garnish with fresh cilantro.
5. Serve with a dollop of Greek yogurt on top.

Nutritional Information per serving: Calories: 450 | Total Fat: 10g | Saturated Fat: 1.5g | Trans Fat: 0g | Polyunsaturated Fat: 2g | Monounsaturated Fat: 5g | Cholesterol: 65mg | Sodium: 300mg | Carbohydrates: 60g | Fiber: 10g | Sugars: 5g | Protein: 35g

Garlic and Herb Turkey Tenderloin

🍴 4 servings   🕐 35 minutes

INGREDIENTS

- 1 turkey tenderloin (about 1.5 lbs)
- 3 cloves garlic, minced
- 2 tablespoons fresh rosemary, chopped
- 2 tablespoons fresh thyme, chopped
- 1 tablespoon olive oil
- 1 tablespoon Dijon mustard
- Salt and black pepper to taste

DIRECTIONS

1. Preheat the oven to 375°F (190°C).
2. In a small bowl, mix together minced garlic, chopped rosemary, chopped thyme, olive oil, Dijon mustard, salt, and black pepper to create the herb mixture.
3. Place the turkey tenderloin in a roasting pan or on a baking sheet.
4. Rub the herb mixture over the turkey tenderloin, ensuring it's evenly coated.
5. Roast in the preheated oven for about 20-25 minutes or until the internal temperature reaches 165°F (74°C) and the turkey is no longer pink in the center.
6. Let the turkey rest for a few minutes before slicing.
7. Serve the garlic and herb turkey tenderloin with your favorite heart-healthy sides.

Nutritional Information per serving: Calories: 200 | Total Fat: 5g | Saturated Fat: 1g | Trans Fat: 0g | Polyunsaturated Fat: 1.5g | Monounsaturated Fat: 2.5g | Cholesterol: 80mg | Sodium: 200mg | Carbohydrates: 1g | Fiber: 0g | Sugars: 0g | Protein: 35g

Lemon Herb Grilled Chicken Breast

🍴 4 servings   🕐 25 minutes

INGREDIENTS

- 4 boneless, skinless chicken breasts
- Zest of 1 lemon
- 3 tablespoons fresh parsley, chopped
- 2 tablespoons fresh thyme, chopped

- 2 tablespoons olive oil
- Juice of 1 lemon
- 2 cloves garlic, minced
- Salt and black pepper to taste

DIRECTIONS

1. Preheat the grill to medium-high heat.
2. In a small bowl, combine lemon zest, chopped parsley, chopped thyme, olive oil, lemon juice, minced garlic, salt, and black pepper to create the marinade.
3. Place the chicken breasts in a shallow dish and coat them with the marinade. Allow them to marinate for at least 30 minutes.
4. Grill the chicken breasts for about 6-8 minutes per side, or until the internal temperature reaches 165°F (74°C) and the chicken is no longer pink in the center.
5. Let the grilled chicken rest for a few minutes before serving.
6. Serve the lemon herb grilled chicken with a side of steamed vegetables or a green salad.

Nutritional Information per serving: Calories: 220 | Total Fat: 9g | Saturated Fat: 1.5g | Trans Fat: 0g | Polyunsaturated Fat: 2g | Monounsaturated Fat: 5g | Cholesterol: 90mg | Sodium: 80mg | Carbohydrates: 2g | Fiber: 0g | Sugars: 0g | Protein: 30g

CHAPTER 7: FISH AND SEAFOOD

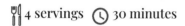

Grilled Salmon with Mango Salsa

🍴 4 servings 🕐 30 minutes

INGREDIENTS

- 4 salmon fillets
- 2 tablespoons olive oil
- Salt and pepper to taste
- For the Mango Salsa:
- 1 ripe mango, diced
- 1/2 red bell pepper, diced
- 1/4 cup red onion, finely chopped
- 1/4 cup fresh cilantro, chopped
- Juice of 1 lime
- Salt to taste

DIRECTIONS

1. Preheat the grill to medium-high heat.
2. Brush salmon fillets with olive oil and season with salt and pepper.
3. Grill salmon for about 5 minutes on each side, or until desired doneness is reached.
4. In a bowl, combine diced mango, red bell pepper, red onion, cilantro, lime juice, and salt to make the salsa.
5. Serve grilled salmon topped with mango salsa.

Nutritional Information per serving: Calories: 310 | Total Fat: 15g | Saturated Fat: 2.5g | Trans Fat: 0g | Polyunsaturated Fat: 4g | Monounsaturated Fat: 8g | Cholesterol: 75mg | Sodium: 120mg | Carbohydrates: 13g | Fiber: 2g | Sugars: 10g | Protein: 31g

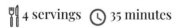

Lemon Pepper Cod with Zucchini Noodles

🍴 4 servings 🕐 35 minutes

INGREDIENTS

- 4 cod fillets
- 2 tablespoons lemon juice
- 1 teaspoon black pepper
- 2 tablespoons olive oil
- 4 zucchini, spiralized into noodles
- 1 clove garlic, minced
- Salt to taste

DIRECTIONS

1. Preheat the oven to 400°F (200°C).
2. Place cod fillets in a baking dish. Drizzle with lemon juice and sprinkle with black pepper.
3. Bake in the preheated oven for 12 minutes, or until fish flakes easily with a fork.
4. While the fish is baking, heat olive oil in a skillet over medium heat. Sauté garlic for 1 minute.
5. Add zucchini noodles to the skillet, cooking for 3-4 minutes or until tender. Season with salt.
6. Serve cod on top of the zucchini noodles.

Nutritional Information per serving: Calories: 220 | Total Fat: 10g | Saturated Fat: 1.5g | Trans Fat: 0g | Polyunsaturated Fat: 1g | Monounsaturated Fat: 7g | Cholesterol: 60mg | Sodium: 90mg | Carbohydrates: 7g | Fiber: 2g | Sugars: 4g | Protein: 26g

Shrimp and Asparagus Stir Fry

🍴 4 servings 🕐 25 minutes

INGREDIENTS

- 1 lb shrimp, peeled and deveined
- 2 cups asparagus, trimmed and cut into pieces
- 2 tablespoons soy sauce (low sodium)
- 1 tablespoon honey
- 1 tablespoon ginger, minced
- 2 cloves garlic, minced
- 1 tablespoon olive oil
- Sesame seeds for garnish

DIRECTIONS

1. In a small bowl, mix together soy sauce, honey, ginger, and garlic.
2. Heat olive oil in a large skillet over medium-high heat.
3. Add asparagus and stir-fry for 2-3 minutes.
4. Add shrimp and stir-fry until they turn pink and are cooked through, about 4-5 minutes.
5. Pour the soy sauce mixture over the shrimp and asparagus. Stir well to coat.
6. Cook for another 2 minutes, then garnish with sesame seeds before serving.

Nutritional Information per serving: Calories: 180 | Total Fat: 6g | Saturated Fat: 1g | Trans Fat: 0g | Polyunsaturated Fat: 1g | Monounsaturated Fat: 3g | Cholesterol: 145mg | Sodium: 480mg | Carbohydrates: 10g | Fiber: 2g | Sugars: 6g | Protein: 24g

Baked Haddock with Herbed Crumbs

🍴 4 servings 🕐 35 minutes

INGREDIENTS
- 4 haddock fillets
- 1 cup whole wheat breadcrumbs
- 1 tablespoon fresh parsley, chopped
- 1 teaspoon fresh thyme, chopped
- 1 clove garlic, minced
- 2 tablespoons olive oil
- Salt and pepper to taste
- Lemon wedges for serving

DIRECTIONS
1. Preheat the oven to 375°F (190°C).
2. In a bowl, mix breadcrumbs, parsley, thyme, garlic, salt, and pepper.
3. Brush each haddock fillet with olive oil, then coat with the breadcrumb mixture.
4. Place fillets on a baking sheet lined with parchment paper.
5. Bake for 20 minutes, or until fish flakes easily with a fork and the crust is golden.
6. Serve with lemon wedges.

Nutritional Information per serving: Calories: 280 | Total Fat: 9g | Saturated Fat: 1.5g | Trans Fat: 0g | Polyunsaturated Fat: 2g | Monounsaturated Fat: 5g | Cholesterol: 85mg | Sodium: 250mg | Carbohydrates: 19g | Fiber: 2g | Sugars: 2g | Protein: 31g

Spicy Tuna and Avocado Cucumber Sushi Rolls

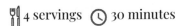

🍴 4 servings 🕐 30 minutes

INGREDIENTS
- 1 cup sushi rice, cooked and cooled
- 8 oz canned tuna, drained
- 1 avocado, thinly sliced
- 1 cucumber, julienned
- 2 tablespoons mayonnaise (low fat)
- 1 teaspoon sriracha sauce
- 4 sheets nori (seaweed)
- Soy sauce (low sodium) for dipping
- Pickled ginger and wasabi for serving

DIRECTIONS
1. In a small bowl, mix together tuna, mayonnaise, and sriracha sauce.
2. Place a sheet of nori on a bamboo sushi mat.
3. Spread a thin layer of sushi rice over the nori, leaving a small margin at the top.
4. Place a line of spicy tuna mixture, avocado slices, and cucumber sticks across the rice.
5. Roll the sushi tightly using the bamboo mat.
6. Cut each roll into 6-8 pieces.
7. Serve with soy sauce, pickled ginger, and wasabi..

Nutritional Information per serving: Calories: 300 | Total Fat: 11g | Saturated Fat: 2g | Trans Fat: 0g | Polyunsaturated Fat: 4g | Monounsaturated Fat: 4g | Cholesterol: 25mg | Sodium: 350mg | Carbohydrates: 33g | Fiber: 4g | Sugars: 2g | Protein: 18g

Seared Scallops with Quinoa and Spinach

🍴 4 servings 🕐 35 minutes

INGREDIENTS
- 12 large sea scallops
- 1 cup quinoa
- 2 cups vegetable broth
- 4 cups fresh spinach
- 2 cloves garlic, minced
- 2 tablespoons olive oil
- Salt and pepper to taste
- Lemon wedges for serving

DIRECTIONS
1. Rinse quinoa under cold water and drain. In a saucepan, bring vegetable broth to a boil. Add quinoa, reduce heat to low, cover, and simmer for 15 minutes, or until liquid is absorbed.
2. While quinoa is cooking, heat 1 tablespoon of olive oil in a skillet over medium-high heat. Season scallops with salt and pepper. Sear scallops for about 2 minutes on each side, or until a golden crust forms. Remove scallops from the skillet and set aside.
3. In the same skillet, add the remaining olive oil and minced garlic. Sauté for 1 minute. Add spinach and cook until wilted.
4. Fluff quinoa with a fork and divide among plates. Top with sautéed spinach and seared scallops.
5. Serve with lemon wedges on the side.

Nutritional Information per serving: Calories: 320 | Total Fat: 10g | Saturated Fat: 1.5g | Trans Fat: 0g | Polyunsaturated Fat: 1g | Monounsaturated Fat: 7g | Cholesterol: 35mg | Sodium: 480mg | Carbohydrates: 36g | Fiber: 4g | Sugars: 1g | Protein: 22g

Mediterranean Shrimp and Orzo Salad

🍴 4 servings   🕐 30 minutes

INGREDIENTS
- 1 cup orzo pasta
- 1 lb shrimp, peeled and deveined
- 2 cups cherry tomatoes, halved
- 1 cucumber, diced
- 1/4 cup Kalamata olives, sliced
- 1/4 cup feta cheese, crumbled
- 1/4 cup red onion, finely chopped
- 1/4 cup fresh parsley, chopped
- 3 tablespoons olive oil
- 2 tablespoons lemon juice
- 1 garlic clove, minced
- Salt and pepper to taste

DIRECTIONS
1. Cook orzo according to package instructions. Drain and let cool.
2. In a skillet, heat 1 tablespoon of olive oil over medium-high heat. Add shrimp, season with salt and pepper, and cook until pink and opaque, about 3-4 minutes per side. Remove from heat.
3. In a large bowl, combine cooked orzo, shrimp, cherry tomatoes, cucumber, olives, feta cheese, red onion, and parsley.
4. In a small bowl, whisk together the remaining olive oil, lemon juice, minced garlic, salt, and pepper to make the dressing.
5. Pour the dressing over the salad and toss to combine.
6. Serve chilled or at room temperature.

Nutritional Information per serving: Calories: 370 | Total Fat: 14g | Saturated Fat: 3g | Trans Fat: 0g | Polyunsaturated Fat: 2g | Monounsaturated Fat: 9g | Cholesterol: 145mg | Sodium: 480mg | Carbohydrates: 39g | Fiber: 3g | Sugars: 5g | Protein: 24g

Teriyaki Glazed Salmon Bowl

🍴 4 servings   🕐 40 minutes

INGREDIENTS
- 4 salmon fillets
- 2 cups cooked brown rice
- 1 broccoli head, cut into florets
- 1 carrot, julienned
- 1 red bell pepper, sliced
- For the Teriyaki Glaze:
- 1/4 cup soy sauce (low sodium)
- 2 tablespoons honey
- 1 tablespoon rice vinegar
- 1 garlic clove, minced
- 1 teaspoon ginger, grated
- 1 tablespoon cornstarch mixed with 2 tablespoons water

DIRECTIONS
1. Preheat the oven to 375°F (190°C). Place salmon fillets on a baking sheet lined with parchment paper.
2. In a small saucepan over medium heat, combine soy sauce, honey, rice vinegar, garlic, and ginger. Bring to a simmer.
3. Stir in the cornstarch and water mixture. Continue to cook, stirring constantly, until the sauce thickens. Remove from heat.
4. Brush salmon fillets with teriyaki glaze and bake for 15-20 minutes, or until cooked through.
5. Meanwhile, steam broccoli florets, julienned carrot, and sliced red bell pepper until tender.
6. Assemble the bowls with brown rice, steamed vegetables, and glazed salmon.
7. Drizzle with additional teriyaki sauce if desired.

Nutritional Information per serving: Calories: 460 | Total Fat: 14g | Saturated Fat: 2.5g | Trans Fat: 0g | Polyunsaturated Fat: 5g | Monounsaturated Fat: 5g | Cholesterol: 60mg | Sodium: 620mg | Carbohydrates: 54g | Fiber: 5g | Sugars: 14g | Protein: 31g

Blackened Tilapia with Cilantro Lime Slaw

🍴 4 servings   🕐 30 minutes

INGREDIENTS
- 4 tilapia fillets
- 2 tablespoons blackening seasoning
- 2 tablespoons olive oil
- For the Slaw:
- 2 cups cabbage, shredded
- 1 carrot, shredded
- 1/4 cup fresh cilantro, chopped
- Juice of 1 lime
- 1 tablespoon honey
- Salt and pepper to taste

DIRECTIONS
1. Season tilapia fillets on both sides with blackening seasoning.
2. Heat olive oil in a skillet over medium-high heat. Cook tilapia for about 3-4 minutes per side, or until cooked through and blackened.
3. In a bowl, combine shredded cabbage, carrot,

cilantro, lime juice, honey, salt, and pepper to make the slaw.
4. Serve blackened tilapia with a side of cilantro lime slaw.

Nutritional Information per serving: Calories: 220 | Total Fat: 9g | Saturated Fat: 1.5g | Trans Fat: 0g | Polyunsaturated Fat: 2g | Monounsaturated Fat: 5g | Cholesterol: 55mg | Sodium: 150mg | Carbohydrates: 12g | Fiber: 2g | Sugars: 8g | Protein: 26g

Seafood Paella with Brown Rice

🍴 6 servings 🕐 1 hour 20 minutes

INGREDIENTS
- 2 cups brown rice
- 4 cups low-sodium chicken or vegetable broth
- 1 lb shrimp, peeled and deveined
- 1/2 lb mussels, cleaned
- 1/2 lb clams, cleaned
- 1 onion, diced
- 1 red bell pepper, sliced
- 2 tomatoes, diced
- 2 cloves garlic, minced
- 1 teaspoon paprika
- 1/2 teaspoon saffron threads
- 2 tablespoons olive oil
- Fresh parsley, chopped for garnish
- Lemon wedges for serving

DIRECTIONS
1. In a large paella pan or skillet, heat olive oil over medium heat. Sauté onion, garlic, and red bell pepper until soft.
2. Add rice and toast for a few minutes. Stir in diced tomatoes, paprika, and saffron.
3. Pour in broth and bring to a simmer. Cook, uncovered, for about 30 minutes, or until rice is almost cooked.
4. Add shrimp, mussels, and clams. Cover and cook for 10 more minutes, or until shellfish open and shrimp are cooked.
5. Garnish with fresh parsley and serve with lemon wedges.

Nutritional Information per serving: Calories: 400 | Total Fat: 10g | Saturated Fat: 1.5g | Trans Fat: 0g | Polyunsaturated Fat: 2g | Monounsaturated Fat: 6g | Cholesterol: 115mg | Sodium: 480mg | Carbohydrates: 54g | Fiber: 4g | Sugars: 4g | Protein: 27g

Crab and Avocado Salad

🍴 4 servings 🕐 15 minutes

INGREDIENTS
- 1 lb crab meat, fresh or canned
- 2 ripe avocados, diced
- 1/4 cup red onion, finely chopped
- 1/4 cup cilantro, chopped
- Juice of 2 limes
- 1 tablespoon olive oil
- Salt and pepper to taste
- Mixed greens for serving

DIRECTIONS
1. In a large bowl, gently combine the crab meat, diced avocados, red onion, and cilantro.
2. In a small bowl, whisk together lime juice, olive oil, salt, and pepper to create a dressing.
3. Pour the dressing over the crab and avocado mixture and toss gently to coat.
4. Serve the salad over a bed of mixed greens.

Nutritional Information per serving: Calories: 260 | Total Fat: 16g | Saturated Fat: 2.5g | Trans Fat: 0g | Polyunsaturated Fat: 2g | Monounsaturated Fat: 10g | Cholesterol: 60mg | Sodium: 480mg | Carbohydrates: 12g | Fiber: 7g | Sugars: 2g | Protein: 20g

Pan-Seared Trout with Almond Butter

🍴 4 servings 🕐 20 minutes

INGREDIENTS
- 4 trout fillets
- 2 tablespoons olive oil
- Salt and pepper to taste
- 1/4 cup almonds, sliced
- 2 tablespoons butter
- 1 lemon, juice and zest
- Fresh parsley, chopped for garnish

DIRECTIONS
1. Season trout fillets with salt and pepper.
2. Heat olive oil in a skillet over medium-high heat. Add trout fillets, skin-side down, and cook for 4-5 minutes. Flip and cook for another 3-4 minutes, or until cooked through.
3. In a separate pan, melt butter over medium heat. Add sliced almonds and cook until golden brown.
4. Stir in lemon juice and zest, then remove from

heat.
5. Drizzle the almond butter sauce over the cooked trout.
6. Garnish with fresh parsley and serve immediately.

Nutritional Information per serving: Calories: 320 | Total Fat: 22g | Saturated Fat: 6g | Trans Fat: 0g | Polyunsaturated Fat: 3g | Monounsaturated Fat: 12g | Cholesterol: 80mg | Sodium: 135mg | Carbohydrates: 3g | Fiber: 1g | Sugars: 1g | Protein: 28g

Miso Soup with Salmon and Bok Choy

🍴 4 servings   🕐 30 minutes

INGREDIENTS

- 4 cups water
- 2 tablespoons miso paste
- 1 lb salmon fillet, cut into chunks
- 2 bok choy, chopped
- 1 carrot, sliced
- 1 tablespoon soy sauce (low sodium)
- 1 teaspoon ginger, grated
- 2 green onions, sliced

DIRECTIONS

1. In a pot, bring water to a simmer. Dissolve miso paste in the water.
2. Add salmon chunks, chopped bok choy, sliced carrot, soy sauce, and grated ginger.
3. Simmer for about 10 minutes, or until the salmon is cooked through and the vegetables are tender.
4. Serve hot, garnished with sliced green onions.

Nutritional Information per serving: Calories: 220 | Total Fat: 9g | Saturated Fat: 1.5g | Trans Fat: 0g | Polyunsaturated Fat: 3.5g | Monounsaturated Fat: 3g | Cholesterol: 55mg | Sodium: 480mg | Carbohydrates: 9g | Fiber: 2g | Sugars: 4g | Protein: 27g

Garlic Lemon Shrimp Skewers

🍴 4 servings   🕐 30 minutes

INGREDIENTS

- 1 lb large shrimp, peeled and deveined
- 3 cloves garlic, minced
- 1 lemon, juice and zest
- 2 tablespoons olive oil
- Salt and pepper to taste
- Wooden skewers, soaked in water

DIRECTIONS

1. In a bowl, combine minced garlic, lemon juice and zest, olive oil, salt, and pepper.
2. Add shrimp to the marinade and let sit for at least 15 minutes in the refrigerator.
3. Thread the marinated shrimp onto soaked skewers.
4. Preheat grill to medium-high heat and grill shrimp skewers for about 3-4 minutes on each side, or until shrimp are pink and opaque.
5. Serve immediately.

Nutritional Information per serving: Calories: 200 | Total Fat: 9g | Saturated Fat: 1.5g | Trans Fat: 0g | Polyunsaturated Fat: 1g | Monounsaturated Fat: 6g | Cholesterol: 145mg | Sodium: 220mg | Carbohydrates: 3g | Fiber: 0g | Sugars: 1g | Protein: 24g

Halibut with Tomato Basil Salsa

🍴 4 servings   🕐 25 minutes

INGREDIENTS

- 4 halibut fillets
- 2 tablespoons olive oil
- Salt and pepper to taste
- For the Tomato Basil Salsa:
- 2 cups cherry tomatoes, halved
- 1/4 cup fresh basil, chopped
- 2 tablespoons red onion, finely chopped
- 1 tablespoon balsamic vinegar
- 1 tablespoon olive oil
- Salt and pepper to taste

DIRECTIONS

1. Preheat the grill to medium-high heat.
2. Brush halibut fillets with olive oil and season with salt and pepper.
3. Grill halibut for about 5 minutes on each side, or until cooked through.
4. In a bowl, mix together cherry tomatoes, basil, red onion, balsamic vinegar, olive oil, salt, and pepper to make the salsa.
5. Serve grilled halibut topped with tomato basil salsa.

Nutritional Information per serving: Calories: 230 | Total Fat: 10g | Saturated Fat: 1.5g | Trans Fat: 0g | Polyunsaturated Fat: 1g | Monounsaturated Fat: 7g | Cholesterol: 55mg | Sodium: 135mg | Carbohydrates: 5g | Fiber: 1g | Sugars: 3g | Protein: 31g

Herb-Crusted Baked Cod

🍴 4 servings   🕐 30 minutes

INGREDIENTS
- 4 cod fillets
- 2 tablespoons olive oil
- 2 tablespoons fresh parsley, chopped
- 1 tablespoon fresh dill, chopped
- 1 tablespoon whole grain mustard
- 1 clove garlic, minced
- Zest of 1 lemon
- Salt and black pepper to taste
- Lemon wedges for serving

DIRECTIONS
1. Preheat the oven to 400°F (200°C).
2. Pat the cod fillets dry with paper towels and place them on a baking sheet lined with parchment paper.
3. In a small bowl, mix together olive oil, chopped parsley, chopped dill, whole grain mustard, minced garlic, lemon zest, salt, and black pepper.
4. Brush the herb mixture over the top of each cod fillet, ensuring an even coating.
5. Bake in the preheated oven for approximately 12-15 minutes or until the fish flakes easily with a fork.
6. Remove the baked cod from the oven and let it rest for a few minutes.
7. Serve the herb-crusted baked cod with a squeeze of fresh lemon juice and your favorite steamed vegetables or a green salad.

Nutritional Information per serving: Calories: 200 | Total Fat: 8g | Saturated Fat: 1g | Trans Fat: 0g | Polyunsaturated Fat: 2g | Monounsaturated Fat: 5g | Cholesterol: 60mg | Sodium: 150mg | Carbohydrates: 1g | Fiber: 0g | Sugars: 0g | Protein: 30g

CHAPTER 8: SNACKS

Baked Sweet Potato Fries with Avocado Dip

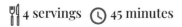 4 servings 🕐 45 minutes

INGREDIENTS
- Ingredients for Sweet Potato Fries:
- 2 large sweet potatoes, peeled and cut into fries
- 2 tablespoons olive oil
- Salt and pepper to taste
- 1 teaspoon paprika
- Ingredients for Avocado Dip:
- 1 ripe avocado
- Juice of 1 lime
- 2 tablespoons Greek yogurt
- Salt and pepper to taste
- 1 clove garlic, minced

DIRECTIONS
1. Preheat the oven to 400°F (200°C). Line a baking sheet with parchment paper.
2. Toss sweet potato fries with olive oil, salt, pepper, and paprika. Spread evenly on the baking sheet.
3. Bake for 30 minutes, turning halfway through, until crispy.
4. For the dip, mash avocado in a bowl. Mix in lime juice, Greek yogurt, salt, pepper, and minced garlic until smooth.
5. Serve the hot sweet potato fries with the avocado dip.

Nutritional Information per serving: Calories: 230 | Total Fat: 14g | Saturated Fat: 2g | Trans Fat: 0g | Polyunsaturated Fat: 2g | Monounsaturated Fat: 10g | Cholesterol: 1mg | Sodium: 120mg | Carbohydrates: 25g | Fiber: 6g | Sugars: 5g | Protein: 3g

Pear and Ricotta Cheese on Multigrain Crackers

🍴 4 servings 🕐 10 minutes

INGREDIENTS
- 4 multigrain crackers
- 1/2 cup ricotta cheese
- 1 ripe pear, thinly sliced
- Honey for drizzling
- Fresh thyme leaves for garnish

DIRECTIONS
1. Spread ricotta cheese evenly over multigrain crackers.
2. Top each cracker with a few slices of pear.
3. Drizzle a small amount of honey over each cracker.
4. Garnish with fresh thyme leaves.
5. Serve immediately as a fresh and satisfying snack.

Nutritional Information per serving: Calories: 150 | Total Fat: 6g | Saturated Fat: 3g | Trans Fat: 0g | Polyunsaturated Fat: 1g | Monounsaturated Fat: 2g | Cholesterol: 20mg | Sodium: 120mg | Carbohydrates: 18g | Fiber: 3g | Sugars: 7g | Protein: 6g

Hummus with Sliced Cucumber and Carrots

🍴 4 servings 🕐 10 minutes

INGREDIENTS
- 2 cups hummus (store-bought or homemade)
- 1 cucumber, sliced
- 2 carrots, peeled and sliced into sticks

DIRECTIONS
1. Arrange hummus in a serving bowl.
2. Surround the bowl with cucumber slices and carrot sticks.
3. Enjoy dipping the fresh vegetables into the hummus for a healthy and crunchy snack.

Nutritional Information per serving: Calories: 150 | Total Fat: 8g | Saturated Fat: 1g | Trans Fat: 0g | Polyunsaturated Fat: 2g | Monounsaturated Fat: 4g | Cholesterol: 0mg | Sodium: 300mg | Carbohydrates: 14g | Fiber: 4g | Sugars: 2g | Protein: 6g

Fresh Fruit Salad with Mint and Lime

🍴 4 servings 🕐 15 minutes

INGREDIENTS
- 2 cups mixed fresh fruit (such as berries, kiwi, mango, and pineapple)
- Juice of 1 lime
- 1 tablespoon honey
- 2 tablespoons fresh mint, chopped

DIRECTIONS

1. In a large bowl, combine the mixed fresh fruit.
2. In a small bowl, whisk together lime juice and honey.
3. Pour the lime-honey dressing over the fruit and toss gently.
4. Sprinkle with chopped mint and toss again lightly.
5. Serve the fruit salad chilled for a refreshing snack.

Nutritional Information per serving: Calories: 90 | Total Fat: 0.5g | Saturated Fat: 0g | Trans Fat: 0g | Polyunsaturated Fat: 0.2g | Monounsaturated Fat: 0.1g | Cholesterol: 0mg | Sodium: 5mg | Carbohydrates: 23g | Fiber: 3g | Sugars: 19g | Protein: 1g

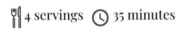

Crispy Baked Zucchini Chips

🍴 4 servings   🕐 35 minutes

INGREDIENTS

- 2 large zucchini, thinly sliced
- 1 tablespoon olive oil
- Salt and pepper to taste
- 1/2 teaspoon paprika (optional)

DIRECTIONS

1. Preheat the oven to 400°F (200°C). Line a baking sheet with parchment paper.
2. In a bowl, toss the zucchini slices with olive oil, salt, pepper, and paprika until evenly coated.
3. Arrange zucchini slices in a single layer on the baking sheet.
4. Bake for 20 minutes or until crisp and golden, flipping halfway through.
5. Let cool before serving as a crunchy, healthy snack.

Nutritional Information per serving: Calories: 60 | Total Fat: 3.5g | Saturated Fat: 0.5g | Trans Fat: 0g | Polyunsaturated Fat: 0.5g | Monounsaturated Fat: 2.5g | Cholesterol: 0mg | Sodium: 75mg | Carbohydrates: 6g | Fiber: 2g | Sugars: 4g | Protein: 2g

Sunflower Seed and Cranberry Energy Bites

🍴 12 bites   🕐 15 minutes

INGREDIENTS

- 1 cup rolled oats
- 1/2 cup sunflower seeds
- 1/4 cup dried cranberries, chopped
- 1/4 cup honey
- 1/2 cup almond butter
- 1 teaspoon vanilla extract

DIRECTIONS

1. In a large bowl, mix together rolled oats, sunflower seeds, and dried cranberries.
2. Add honey, almond butter, and vanilla extract to the mixture. Stir until well combined.
3. Using your hands, roll the mixture into bite-sized balls.
4. Place the energy bites in the refrigerator for at least 1 hour to set.
5. Enjoy as a healthy, energy-boosting snack.

Nutritional Information per bite: Calories: 140 | Total Fat: 8g | Saturated Fat: 1g | Trans Fat: 0g | Polyunsaturated Fat: 3g | Monounsaturated Fat: 4g | Cholesterol: 0mg | Sodium: 15mg | Carbohydrates: 15g | Fiber: 2g | Sugars: 7g | Protein: 4g

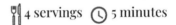

Whole Grain Rice Cakes with Almond Butter and Berries

🍴 4 servings   🕐 5 minutes

INGREDIENTS

- 4 whole grain rice cakes
- 4 tablespoons almond butter
- 1 cup mixed berries (such as strawberries, blueberries, raspberries)
- Honey for drizzling (optional)

DIRECTIONS

1. Spread 1 tablespoon of almond butter on each rice cake.
2. Top each rice cake with a mix of berries.
3. Optionally, drizzle a small amount of honey over each rice cake.
4. Serve immediately as a nutritious snack.

Nutritional Information per serving: Calories: 180 | Total Fat: 8g | Saturated Fat: 1g | Trans Fat: 0g | Polyunsaturated Fat: 2g | Monounsaturated Fat: 4g | Cholesterol: 0mg | Sodium: 60mg | Carbohydrates: 24g | Fiber: 4g | Sugars: 7g | Protein: 5g

Spinach and Feta Stuffed Mushrooms

🍴 4 servings 🕐 25 minutes

INGREDIENTS

- 12 large button mushrooms, stems removed
- 2 cups spinach, chopped
- 1/2 cup feta cheese, crumbled
- 2 cloves garlic, minced
- 2 tablespoons olive oil
- Salt and pepper to taste

DIRECTIONS

1. Preheat the oven to 375°F (190°C). Line a baking sheet with parchment paper.
2. In a skillet, heat 1 tablespoon of olive oil over medium heat. Sauté garlic and spinach until the spinach is wilted.
3. Remove from heat and stir in feta cheese. Season with salt and pepper.
4. Stuff each mushroom cap with the spinach and feta mixture.
5. Place the stuffed mushrooms on the baking sheet. Drizzle with the remaining olive oil.
6. Bake for 20 minutes or until the mushrooms are tender.
7. Serve warm as a delicious and healthy appetizer.

Nutritional Information per serving: Calories: 120 | Total Fat: 9g | Saturated Fat: 3g | Trans Fat: 0g | Polyunsaturated Fat: 1g | Monounsaturated Fat: 5g | Cholesterol: 15mg | Sodium: 250mg | Carbohydrates: 6g | Fiber: 1g | Sugars: 3g | Protein: 5g

Cucumber Boats Filled with Tuna Salad

🍴 4 servings 🕐 15 minutes

INGREDIENTS

- 2 large cucumbers
- 1 can (5 oz) tuna in water, drained
- 1/4 cup Greek yogurt
- 2 tablespoons red onion, finely chopped
- 1 tablespoon fresh dill, chopped
- 1 tablespoon lemon juice
- Salt and pepper to taste

DIRECTIONS

1. Cut the cucumbers in half lengthwise and scoop out the seeds to create boats.
2. In a bowl, mix together tuna, Greek yogurt, red onion, dill, and lemon juice. Season with salt and pepper.
3. Spoon the tuna mixture into the cucumber boats.
4. Serve chilled as a refreshing and healthy snack.

Nutritional Information per serving: Calories: 100 | Total Fat: 2g | Saturated Fat: 0.5g | Trans Fat: 0g | Polyunsaturated Fat: 0.5g | Monounsaturated Fat: 0.5g | Cholesterol: 15mg | Sodium: 170mg | Carbohydrates: 6g | Fiber: 1g | Sugars: 3g | Protein: 14g

CHAPTER 9: DESSERT

Carrot and Walnut Cake with Greek Yogurt Frosting

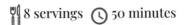 8 servings 🕐 50 minutes

INGREDIENTS
- Ingredients for Cake:
- 2 cups whole wheat flour
- 2 teaspoons baking powder
- 1 teaspoon baking soda
- 1 teaspoon cinnamon
- 1/2 teaspoon nutmeg
- 1/4 teaspoon salt
- 3/4 cup honey or maple syrup
- 1/2 cup unsweetened applesauce
- 1/4 cup olive oil
- 2 eggs
- 2 cups grated carrots
- 1/2 cup walnuts, chopped
- Ingredients for Frosting:
- 1 cup Greek yogurt
- 2 tablespoons honey
- 1 teaspoon vanilla extract

DIRECTIONS
1. Preheat the oven to 350°F (175°C). Grease a 9-inch cake pan.
2. In a bowl, mix flour, baking powder, baking soda, cinnamon, nutmeg, and salt.
3. In another bowl, whisk together honey, applesauce, olive oil, and eggs.
4. Gradually add the dry ingredients to the wet ingredients, mixing until just combined.
5. Fold in the grated carrots and walnuts.
6. Pour the batter into the prepared pan and bake for 30 minutes, or until a toothpick comes out clean.
7. For the frosting, whisk together Greek yogurt, honey, and vanilla.
8. Once the cake is cool, spread the Greek yogurt frosting over the top.
9. Serve and enjoy!

Nutritional Information per serving: Calories: 350 | Total Fat: 12g | Saturated Fat: 2g | Trans Fat: 0g | Polyunsaturated Fat: 3g | Monounsaturated Fat: 6g | Cholesterol: 45mg | Sodium: 250mg | Carbohydrates: 55g | Fiber: 5g | Sugars: 30g | Protein: 8g

No-Bake Date and Nut Energy Balls

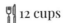 12 balls 🕐 15 minutes

INGREDIENTS
- 1 cup dates, pitted
- 1/2 cup almonds
- 1/2 cup walnuts
- 1/4 cup unsweetened shredded coconut
- 1 tablespoon chia seeds
- 1 teaspoon vanilla extract

DIRECTIONS
1. In a food processor, blend dates, almonds, walnuts, shredded coconut, chia seeds, and vanilla extract until a sticky dough forms.
2. Roll the mixture into 12 small balls.
3. Place the energy balls in the refrigerator for at least 1 hour to firm up.
4. Enjoy as a healthy, energy-boosting snack.

Nutritional Information per ball: Calories: 110 | Total Fat: 7g | Saturated Fat: 1.5g | Trans Fat: 0g | Polyunsaturated Fat: 2.5g | Monounsaturated Fat: 2.5g | Cholesterol: 0mg | Sodium: 0mg | Carbohydrates: 12g | Fiber: 2g | Sugars: 8g | Protein: 2g

Pumpkin Spice Baked Oatmeal Cups

🍴 12 cups 🕐 30 minutes

INGREDIENTS
- 3 cups rolled oats
- 1 teaspoon baking powder
- 2 teaspoons pumpkin pie spice
- 1/4 teaspoon salt
- 1 cup pumpkin puree
- 1/4 cup honey or maple syrup
- 2 eggs
- 1 1/2 cups milk (almond or cow's)
- 1/2 cup raisins or chopped nuts (optional)

DIRECTIONS
1. Preheat the oven to 350°F (175°C). Grease a 12-cup muffin tin.

2. In a large bowl, mix together oats, baking powder, pumpkin pie spice, and salt.
3. In another bowl, combine pumpkin puree, honey, eggs, and milk.
4. Add the wet ingredients to the dry ingredients and stir to combine. Fold in raisins or nuts if using.
5. Divide the mixture evenly among the muffin cups.
6. Bake for 20 minutes, or until the tops are set and golden.
7. Allow to cool before serving.

Nutritional Information per cup: Calories: 140 | Total Fat: 3g | Saturated Fat: 0.5g | Trans Fat: 0g | Polyunsaturated Fat: 1g | Monounsaturated Fat: 1g | Cholesterol: 30mg | Sodium: 80mg | Carbohydrates: 24g | Fiber: 3g | Sugars: 9g | Protein: 5g

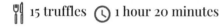

Dark Chocolate Avocado Truffles

🍴 15 truffles 🕐 1 hour 20 minutes

INGREDIENTS
- 2 ripe avocados, mashed
- 1 cup dark chocolate, melted
- 2 tablespoons cocoa powder
- 1 tablespoon honey
- 1/4 teaspoon vanilla extract
- Pinch of salt
- Additional cocoa powder for coating

DIRECTIONS
1. In a bowl, combine mashed avocados, melted dark chocolate, cocoa powder, honey, vanilla extract, and a pinch of salt. Mix until smooth.
2. Refrigerate the mixture for 30 minutes to firm up.
3. Using a spoon, scoop out small portions of the mixture and roll into balls.
4. Roll each truffle in additional cocoa powder to coat.
5. Place truffles in the refrigerator for an additional 30 minutes to set.
6. Enjoy a decadent, heart-healthy treat.

Nutritional Information per truffle: Calories: 100 | Total Fat: 7g | Saturated Fat: 3g | Trans Fat: 0g | Polyunsaturated Fat: 0.5g | Monounsaturated Fat: 3g | Cholesterol: 0mg | Sodium: 10mg | Carbohydrates: 10g | Fiber: 2g | Sugars: 6g | Protein: 1g

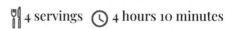

Raspberry and Lemon Chia Pudding

🍴 4 servings 🕐 4 hours 10 minutes

INGREDIENTS
- 1/4 cup chia seeds
- 1 cup unsweetened almond milk
- 1/2 cup Greek yogurt
- 2 tablespoons honey or maple syrup
- Juice and zest of 1 lemon
- 1 cup fresh raspberries

DIRECTIONS
1. In a bowl, whisk together almond milk, Greek yogurt, honey, lemon juice, and lemon zest.
2. Stir in the chia seeds.
3. Gently fold in the raspberries.
4. Divide the mixture into four serving glasses or bowls.
5. Refrigerate for at least 4 hours, or overnight, until the pudding is set.
6. Serve chilled, garnished with additional raspberries or lemon zest if desired.

Nutritional Information per serving: Calories: 150 | Total Fat: 5g | Saturated Fat: 0.5g | Trans Fat: 0g | Polyunsaturated Fat: 3g | Monounsaturated Fat: 1g | Cholesterol: 3mg | Sodium: 45mg | Carbohydrates: 21g | Fiber: 7g | Sugars: 11g | Protein: 6g

Pear and Ginger Crumble

🍴 6 servings 🕐 45 minutes

INGREDIENTS
- 4 ripe pears, peeled and sliced
- 1 tablespoon fresh ginger, grated
- 1/2 cup rolled oats
- 1/4 cup almond flour
- 1/4 cup walnuts, chopped
- 2 tablespoons coconut oil, melted
- 2 tablespoons honey or maple syrup
- 1 teaspoon cinnamon

DIRECTIONS
1. Preheat the oven to 350°F (175°C).
2. Place the pear slices in a baking dish and sprinkle with grated ginger.
3. In a bowl, combine rolled oats, almond flour, chopped walnuts, melted coconut oil, honey, and

cinnamon. Mix until crumbly.
4. Sprinkle the oat mixture over the pears.
5. Bake for 30 minutes, or until the topping is golden and the pears are tender.
6. Serve warm, possibly with a dollop of Greek yogurt or a drizzle of honey.

Nutritional Information per serving: Calories: 200 | Total Fat: 10g | Saturated Fat: 4g | Trans Fat: 0g | Polyunsaturated Fat: 2g | Monounsaturated Fat: 3g | Cholesterol: 0mg | Sodium: 5mg | Carbohydrates: 27g | Fiber: 5g | Sugars: 15g | Protein: 3g

Coconut and Almond Macaroons (Sugar-Free)

🍴 15 macaroons   🕐 25 minutes

INGREDIENTS
- 2 cups unsweetened shredded coconut
- 1 cup almond flour
- 1/4 cup coconut oil, melted
- 1/4 cup honey or maple syrup
- 1 teaspoon almond extract
- 2 egg whites

DIRECTIONS
1. Preheat the oven to 350°F (175°C). Line a baking sheet with parchment paper.
2. In a bowl, combine shredded coconut, almond flour, melted coconut oil, honey, and almond extract.
3. In another bowl, beat the egg whites until stiff peaks form.
4. Gently fold the egg whites into the coconut mixture.
5. Using a spoon or cookie scoop, form the mixture into small mounds on the prepared baking sheet.
6. Bake for 15 minutes, or until the macaroons are golden.
7. Let cool before serving.

Nutritional Information per macaroon: Calories: 140 | Total Fat: 12g | Saturated Fat: 8g | Trans Fat: 0g | Polyunsaturated Fat: 0.5g | Monounsaturated Fat: 2g | Cholesterol: 0mg | Sodium: 15mg | Carbohydrates: 8g | Fiber: 2g | Sugars: 5g | Protein: 3g

Flourless Black Bean Brownies

🍴 12 brownies   🕐 35 minutes

INGREDIENTS
- 1 can (15 oz) black beans, drained and rinsed
- 3 eggs
- 1/3 cup coconut oil, melted
- 1/4 cup cocoa powder
- 2 teaspoons vanilla extract
- 1/2 cup honey or maple syrup
- 1/2 teaspoon baking powder
- Pinch of salt
- 1/2 cup dark chocolate chips (optional)

DIRECTIONS
1. Preheat the oven to 350°F (175°C). Grease an 8-inch square baking pan.
2. In a food processor, blend black beans, eggs, melted coconut oil, cocoa powder, vanilla extract, honey, baking powder, and salt until smooth.
3. Stir in chocolate chips, if using.
4. Pour the batter into the prepared baking pan.
5. Bake for 25 minutes, or until the brownies are set and a toothpick comes out clean.
6. Let cool before cutting into squares.

Nutritional Information per brownie: Calories: 180 | Total Fat: 10g | Saturated Fat: 7g | Trans Fat: 0g | Polyunsaturated Fat: 0.5g | Monounsaturated Fat: 2g | Cholesterol: 45mg | Sodium: 75mg | Carbohydrates: 20g | Fiber: 3g | Sugars: 14g | Protein: 4g

Zucchini and Chocolate Chip Muffins

🍴 12 muffins   🕐 35 minutes

INGREDIENTS
- 1 1/2 cups whole wheat flour
- 1 teaspoon baking powder
- 1/2 teaspoon baking soda
- 1 teaspoon cinnamon
- 1/2 cup honey or maple syrup
- 1/2 cup unsweetened applesauce
- 1 egg
- 1 teaspoon vanilla extract
- 1 cup zucchini, grated
- 1/2 cup dark chocolate chips

DIRECTIONS
1. Preheat the oven to 350°F (175°C). Line a muffin tin with paper liners.
2. In a bowl, mix together flour, baking powder, baking soda, and cinnamon.
3. In another bowl, whisk together honey, applesauce, egg, and vanilla extract.
4. Add the wet ingredients to the dry ingredients and mix until just combined.
5. Fold in grated zucchini and chocolate chips.

6.Divide the batter evenly among the muffin cups.

7.Bake for 20 minutes, or until a toothpick comes out clean.

8.Let cool before serving.

Nutritional Information per muffin: Calories: 180 | Total Fat: 4g | Saturated Fat: 2g | Trans Fat: 0g | Polyunsaturated Fat: 0.5g | Monounsaturated Fat: 1g | Cholesterol: 15mg | Sodium: 100mg | Carbohydrates: 34g | Fiber: 3g | Sugars: 18g | Protein: 3g

CHAPTER 10: SMOOTHIES AND MOCKTAILS

Carrot Ginger Turmeric Smoothie
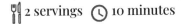

🍴 2 servings 🕐 10 minutes

INGREDIENTS
- 2 large carrots, peeled and chopped
- 1 ripe banana
- 1/2 inch fresh ginger, peeled and minced
- 1/2 teaspoon ground turmeric
- 1 tablespoon honey (optional)
- 1 cup almond milk or water
- Ice cubes (optional)

DIRECTIONS
1. In a blender, combine the chopped carrots, banana, ginger, turmeric, honey (if using), and almond milk or water.
2. Blend until smooth. If the smoothie is too thick, add a little more liquid to reach the desired consistency.
3. Add ice cubes if you prefer a colder smoothie.
4. Blend again until the ice is fully incorporated.
5. Serve immediately for a refreshing and nutritious drink.

Nutritional Information per serving: Calories: 120 | Total Fat: 1.5g | Saturated Fat: 0g | Trans Fat: 0g | Polyunsaturated Fat: 0.5g | Monounsaturated Fat: 0.5g | Cholesterol: 0mg | Sodium: 80mg | Carbohydrates: 26g | Fiber: 4g | Sugars: 16g (including honey) | Protein: 2g

Beetroot and Pomegranate Smoothie

🍴 2 servings 🕐 10 minutes

INGREDIENTS
- 1 medium beetroot, cooked and peeled
- 1/2 cup pomegranate seeds
- 1 apple, cored and sliced
- 1/2 cup Greek yogurt
- 1 cup water or coconut water
- Ice cubes (optional)

DIRECTIONS
1. In a blender, combine cooked beetroot, pomegranate seeds, apple slices, Greek yogurt, and water or coconut water.
2. Blend until smooth. Add ice cubes if desired for a colder smoothie.
3. Blend again until all ingredients are well combined.
4. Serve immediately, enjoying the antioxidant-rich and heart-healthy benefits.

Nutritional Information per serving: Calories: 150 | Total Fat: 1g | Saturated Fat: 0g | Trans Fat: 0g | Polyunsaturated Fat: 0g | Monounsaturated Fat: 0g | Cholesterol: 5mg | Sodium: 55mg | Carbohydrates: 30g | Fiber: 5g | Sugars: 22g | Protein: 7g

Spinach, Kiwi, and Flaxseed Smoothie

🍴 2 servings 🕐 10 minutes

INGREDIENTS
- 2 cups fresh spinach
- 2 ripe kiwis, peeled and sliced
- 1 tablespoon ground flaxseed
- 1 ripe banana
- 1 cup unsweetened almond milk
- Ice cubes (optional)

DIRECTIONS
1. In a blender, combine spinach, kiwi slices, ground flaxseed, banana, and almond milk.
2. Blend until smooth. If the smoothie is too thick, add a little more almond milk.
3. Add ice cubes if you prefer a colder smoothie.
4. Blend again until the ice is fully incorporated.
5. Serve immediately for a nutrient-packed and energizing drink.

Nutritional Information per serving: Calories: 130 | Total Fat: 3g | Saturated Fat: 0g | Trans Fat: 0g | Polyunsaturated Fat: 1.5g | Monounsaturated Fat: 0.5g | Cholesterol: 0mg | Sodium: 95mg | Carbohydrates: 24g | Fiber: 5g | Sugars: 12g | Protein: 3g

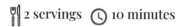

Pineapple and Coconut Water Hydration Smoothie

🍴 2 servings 🕐 10 minutes

INGREDIENTS

- 2 cups fresh pineapple, cubed
- 1 cup coconut water
- 1/2 banana
- Juice of 1 lime
- Ice cubes (optional)

DIRECTIONS

1. In a blender, combine pineapple cubes, coconut water, banana, and lime juice.
2. Blend until smooth. If the smoothie is too thick, add a little more coconut water.
3. Add ice cubes if you prefer a colder smoothie.
4. Blend again until the ice is fully incorporated.
5. Serve immediately for a hydrating and refreshing tropical drink.

Nutritional Information per serving: Calories: 100 | Total Fat: 0.5g | Saturated Fat: 0g | Trans Fat: 0g | Polyunsaturated Fat: 0g | Monounsaturated Fat: 0g | Cholesterol: 0mg | Sodium: 65mg | Carbohydrates: 25g | Fiber: 3g | Sugars: 18g | Protein: 2g

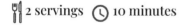

Cucumber, Lime, and Mint Green Smoothie

🍴 2 servings 🕐 10 minutes

INGREDIENTS

- 1 large cucumber, chopped
- Juice of 2 limes
- 1/4 cup fresh mint leaves
- 1 cup fresh spinach
- 1 green apple, cored and sliced
- 1 tablespoon honey (optional)
- 1 cup water or coconut water
- Ice cubes (optional)

DIRECTIONS

1. In a blender, combine the cucumber, lime juice, mint leaves, spinach, green apple, and honey if desired.
2. Add water or coconut water for a smoother consistency.
3. Blend until smooth. Add ice cubes for a chilled smoothie, if you like.
4. Blend again until the ice is fully integrated.
5. Serve immediately for a refreshing and hydrating beverage.

Nutritional Information per serving: Calories: 80 | Total Fat: 0.5g | Saturated Fat: 0g | Trans Fat: 0g | Polyunsaturated Fat: 0.2g | Monounsaturated Fat: 0.1g | Cholesterol: 0mg | Sodium: 25mg | Carbohydrates: 20g | Fiber: 3g | Sugars: 14g | Protein: 2g

Sparkling Cranberry and Lime Mocktail

🍴 4 servings 🕐 5 minutes

INGREDIENTS

- 2 cups cranberry juice, unsweetened
- Juice of 2 limes
- 2 cups sparkling water
- Ice cubes
- Fresh cranberries and lime slices for garnish

DIRECTIONS

1. In a pitcher, mix together cranberry juice and lime juice.
2. Just before serving, add sparkling water to the juice mixture.
3. Fill glasses with ice cubes and pour the mocktail over the ice.
4. Garnish with fresh cranberries and lime slices.
5. Serve immediately for a fizzy and tangy drink.

Nutritional Information per serving: Calories: 60 | Total Fat: 0g | Saturated Fat: 0g | Trans Fat: 0g | Polyunsaturated Fat: 0g | Monounsaturated Fat: 0g | Cholesterol: 0mg | Sodium: 10mg | Carbohydrates: 15g | Fiber: 0g | Sugars: 14g | Protein: 0g

Watermelon and Basil Refresher

🍴 4 servings 🕐 10 minutes

INGREDIENTS

- 4 cups watermelon, cubed and seeds removed
- 1/4 cup fresh basil leaves
- Juice of 1 lime
- 1 tablespoon honey (optional)
- 2 cups ice cubes
- Sparkling water for topping

DIRECTIONS

1. In a blender, combine watermelon, basil leaves, lime juice, and honey if using. Blend until smooth.
2. Strain the mixture through a fine mesh sieve into a pitcher.

3. Fill glasses with ice cubes and pour the watermelon mixture over the ice, filling each glass about two-thirds full.
4. Top each glass with sparkling water.
5. Stir gently and serve immediately for a cooling and aromatic drink.

Nutritional Information per serving: Calories: 50 | Total Fat: 0.2g | Saturated Fat: 0g | Trans Fat: 0g | Polyunsaturated Fat: 0.1g | Monounsaturated Fat: 0.1g | Cholesterol: 0mg | Sodium: 5mg | Carbohydrates: 12g | Fiber: 1g | Sugars: 10g | Protein: 1g

Non-Alcoholic Sangria with Mixed Berries

🍴 6 servings 🕐 1 hour 10 minutes

INGREDIENTS
- 3 cups mixed berries (strawberries, blueberries, raspberries)
- Juice of 2 oranges
- Juice of 1 lemon
- 2 cinnamon sticks
- 3 cups grape juice, unsweetened
- 2 cups sparkling water
- Ice cubes
- Orange and lemon slices for garnish

DIRECTIONS
1. In a large pitcher, combine mixed berries, orange juice, lemon juice, and cinnamon sticks.
2. Add grape juice and stir well.
3. Refrigerate for at least 1 hour to allow the flavors to blend.
4. Just before serving, add sparkling water and stir gently.
5. Serve over ice cubes, garnished with orange and lemon slices.

Nutritional Information per serving: Calories: 120 | Total Fat: 0.5g | Saturated Fat: 0g | Trans Fat: 0g | Polyunsaturated Fat: 0.2g | Monounsaturated Fat: 0.1g | Cholesterol: 0mg | Sodium: 25mg | Carbohydrates: 30g | Fiber: 2g | Sugars: 25g | Protein: 1g

Lavender and Honey Sparkling Lemonade

🍴 4 servings 🕐 1 hour 15 minutes

INGREDIENTS

- 4 cups water
- 2 tablespoons dried lavender flowers (culinary grade)
- 1/3 cup honey (or to taste)
- 3/4 cup fresh lemon juice (about 4-5 lemons)
- 2 cups sparkling water
- Ice cubes
- Lemon slices and fresh lavender sprigs for garnish

DIRECTIONS
1. In a saucepan, bring 1 cup of water to a boil. Remove from heat and add the lavender flowers. Let steep for 5 minutes.
2. Strain the lavender-infused water into a pitcher, discarding the lavender flowers.
3. Stir in the honey until dissolved.
4. Add the remaining 3 cups of water and lemon juice to the pitcher. Mix well.
5. Refrigerate the lemonade until chilled, about 1 hour.
6. Just before serving, stir in the sparkling water.
7. Serve over ice, garnished with lemon slices and lavender sprigs.

Nutritional Information per serving: Calories: 60 | Total Fat: 0g | Saturated Fat: 0g | Trans Fat: 0g | Polyunsaturated Fat: 0g | Monounsaturated Fat: 0g | Cholesterol: 0mg | Sodium: 10mg | Carbohydrates: 17g | Fiber: 0g | Sugars: 15g | Protein: 0g

Virgin Mojito with Fresh Mint and Lime

🍴 4 servings 🕐 10 minutes

INGREDIENTS
- 1/2 cup fresh mint leaves
- 2 limes, juiced
- 2 tablespoons honey or agave syrup
- 4 cups sparkling water or club soda
- Ice cubes
- Extra mint sprigs and lime slices for garnish

DIRECTIONS
1. In a pitcher, muddle the mint leaves with lime juice and honey or agave syrup to release the mint flavors.
2. Add the sparkling water or club soda to the pitcher and stir gently.
3. Fill glasses with ice and pour the mojito mixture over the ice.
4. Garnish each glass with a sprig of mint and a slice of lime.
5. Serve immediately for a refreshing and zesty mocktail.

Nutritional Information per serving: Calories: 40 | Total Fat: 0g | Saturated Fat: 0g | Trans Fat: 0g | Polyunsaturated Fat: 0g | Monounsaturated Fat: 0g | Cholesterol: 0mg | Sodium: 10mg | Carbohydrates: 11g | Fiber: 1g | Sugars: 8g | Protein: 0g

CHAPTER 11: BONUS: AIR FRYER RECIPES

Crispy Quinoa Patties with Lemon Herb Yogurt Sauce

🍴 4 servings 🕐 35 minutes

INGREDIENTS

- 1 cup cooked quinoa, cooled
- 1/2 cup whole-grain breadcrumbs
- 1/4 cup finely grated Parmesan cheese
- 1/4 cup finely chopped red bell pepper
- 2 green onions, finely chopped
- 2 cloves garlic, minced
- 1 large egg, beaten
- 1 tablespoon olive oil
- 1 teaspoon dried oregano
- 1/2 teaspoon smoked paprika
- Cooking spray
- 1/2 cup Greek yogurt (low-fat or fat-free)
- Zest of 1 lemon
- 1 tablespoon lemon juice
- 2 tablespoons fresh parsley, finely chopped
- 1 tablespoon fresh dill, finely chopped
- Salt and pepper to taste

DIRECTIONS

1. In a large mixing bowl, combine cooked quinoa, breadcrumbs, Parmesan cheese, red bell pepper, green onions, garlic, beaten egg, olive oil, oregano, smoked paprika, salt, and pepper.
2. Mix the ingredients until well combined. If the mixture is too wet, add more breadcrumbs; if too dry, add a splash of water.
3. Form the mixture into patties, about 2-3 inches in diameter.
4. Preheat your air fryer to 375°F (190°C).
5. Lightly coat the quinoa patties with cooking spray.
6. Place the patties in the air fryer basket, leaving space between each.
7. Air fry for 18-20 minutes, flipping halfway through, until the patties are golden brown and crispy.
8. In a small bowl, mix together Greek yogurt, lemon zest, lemon juice, chopped parsley, chopped dill, salt, and pepper.
9. Adjust seasoning according to taste.
10. Serve the crispy quinoa patties with a dollop of lemon herb yogurt sauce on top.

Nutritional Information per serving: Calories: 220 | Total Fat: 8g | Saturated Fat: 2g | Trans Fat: 0g | Polyunsaturated Fat: 1.5g | Monounsaturated Fat: 4g | Cholesterol: 55mg | Sodium: 250mg | Carbohydrates: 26g | Fiber: 4g | Sugars: 2g | Protein: 11g

Sweet Potato and Chickpea Falafel Bowls with Tahini Drizzle

🍴 4 servings 🕐 35 minutes

INGREDIENTS

- 1 can (15 oz) chickpeas, drained and rinsed
- 1 large sweet potato, peeled and grated
- 1/4 cup red onion, finely chopped
- 2 cloves garlic, minced
- 1 teaspoon ground cumin
- 1 teaspoon ground coriander
- 1/2 teaspoon smoked paprika
- 2 tablespoons whole wheat flour or chickpea flour
- 1 tablespoon olive oil (for brushing)
- 1/4 cup tahini
- 2 tablespoons lemon juice
- 2 tablespoons water
- 1 clove garlic, minced
- Whole grain or quinoa, cooked
- Cherry tomatoes, halved
- Cucumber, sliced
- Red onion, thinly sliced
- Fresh parsley, chopped
- Salt and pepper to taste

DIRECTIONS

1. Preheat the air fryer to 375°F (190°C).
2. In a food processor, combine chickpeas, grated sweet potato, red onion, garlic, cumin, coriander, smoked paprika, flour, salt, and pepper.
3. Pulse until the mixture comes together but still has some texture.
4. Form the mixture into falafel patties and brush each with olive oil.
5. Place the falafel in the air fryer basket, leaving space between each.
6. Air fry for 12-15 minutes, flipping halfway through, until the falafel are golden brown and cooked through.

7. In a bowl, whisk together tahini, lemon juice, water, minced garlic, and salt. Adjust the consistency with more water if needed.
8. Assemble the bowls with cooked whole grain or quinoa, cherry tomatoes, cucumber slices, red onion slices, and fresh parsley.
9. Top the bowls with the air-fried sweet potato and chickpea falafel.
10. Drizzle with tahini sauce before serving.

Nutritional Information per serving: Calories: 280 | Total Fat: 16g | Saturated Fat: 2g | Trans Fat: 0g | Polyunsaturated Fat: 5g | Monounsaturated Fat: 8g | Cholesterol: 0mg | Sodium: 260mg | Carbohydrates: 30g | Fiber: 8g | Sugars: 5g | Protein: 8g

Balsamic Glazed Brussels Sprouts with Toasted Almonds

🍴 4 servings   🕐 25 minutes

INGREDIENTS
- 1 pound Brussels sprouts, trimmed and halved
- 2 tablespoons balsamic vinegar
- 1 tablespoon olive oil
- 1 tablespoon maple syrup
- Salt and pepper to taste
- 1/4 cup almonds, sliced and toasted

DIRECTIONS
1. In a bowl, toss Brussels sprouts with balsamic vinegar, olive oil, maple syrup, salt, and pepper until well coated.
2. Preheat the air fryer to 375°F (190°C).
3. Place the Brussels sprouts in the air fryer basket, spreading them out for even cooking.
4. Air fry for 12-15 minutes, shaking the basket halfway through, until Brussels sprouts are caramelized and crispy on the edges.
5. While the Brussels sprouts are cooking, toast the sliced almonds in a dry pan over medium heat until golden brown. Keep a close eye to prevent burning.
6. Once the Brussels sprouts are done, transfer them to a serving dish and sprinkle with toasted almonds.

Nutritional Information per serving: Calories: 120 | Total Fat: 7g | Saturated Fat: 1g | Trans Fat: 0g | Polyunsaturated Fat: 2g | Monounsaturated Fat: 4g | Cholesterol: 0mg | Sodium: 25mg | Carbohydrates: 14g | Fiber: 4g | Sugars: 6g | Protein: 4g

Turmeric Spiced Cauliflower Bites with Mint Yogurt Dip

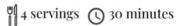

🍴 4 servings   🕐 30 minutes

INGREDIENTS
- 1 medium cauliflower, cut into florets
- 2 tablespoons olive oil
- 1 teaspoon ground turmeric
- 1/2 teaspoon ground cumin
- 1/2 teaspoon smoked paprika
- 1/2 cup Greek yogurt (low-fat or fat-free)
- 2 tablespoons fresh mint, chopped
- 1 tablespoon lemon juice
- Salt and pepper to taste

DIRECTIONS
1. In a large bowl, toss cauliflower florets with olive oil, turmeric, cumin, smoked paprika, salt, and pepper until evenly coated.
2. Preheat the air fryer to 375°F (190°C).
3. Place the cauliflower in the air fryer basket, spreading them out for even cooking.
4. Air fry for 12-15 minutes, shaking the basket halfway through, until the cauliflower is golden brown and crispy.
5. In a small bowl, mix together Greek yogurt, chopped mint, lemon juice, salt, and pepper.
6. Adjust seasoning to taste.
7. Serve the Turmeric Spiced Cauliflower Bites with Mint Yogurt Dip.

Nutritional Information per serving: Calories:120 | Total Fat: 7g | Saturated Fat: 1g | Trans Fat: 0g | Polyunsaturated Fat: 1g | Monounsaturated Fat: 5g | Cholesterol: 1mg | Sodium: 30mg | Carbohydrates: 14g | Fiber: 5g | Sugars: 5g | Protein: 6g

Mango and Jalapeño Turkey Burger Sliders

🍴 8 sliders   🕐 30 minutes

INGREDIENTS
- 1 pound lean ground turkey
- 1/2 cup mango, finely diced
- 1 jalapeño, seeds removed and finely diced
- 2 green onions, finely chopped
- 1 clove garlic, minced
- 1 teaspoon ground cumin
- 1 teaspoon chili powder
- Salt and pepper to taste
- Whole grain slider buns

- Lettuce leaves
- Sliced tomatoes

DIRECTIONS

1. In a bowl, combine ground turkey, diced mango, diced jalapeño, chopped green onions, minced garlic, ground cumin, chili powder, salt, and pepper. Mix until well combined.
2. Shape the mixture into small slider-sized patties.
3. Preheat the air fryer to 375°F (190°C).
4. Place the turkey patties in the air fryer basket, ensuring they are not touching, and air fry for 12-15 minutes or until the internal temperature reaches 165°F (74°C), flipping halfway through.
5. Assemble sliders with lettuce, turkey patties, and sliced tomatoes on whole grain slider buns.

Nutritional Information per serving: Calories: 280 | Total Fat: 8g | Saturated Fat: 2g | Trans Fat: 0g | Polyunsaturated Fat: 2g | Monounsaturated Fat: 3g | Cholesterol: 80mg | Sodium: 220mg | Carbohydrates: 26g | Fiber: 4g | Sugars: 6g | Protein: 26g

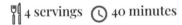

Mediterranean Eggplant and Chickpea Stacks

🍴 4 servings 🕐 40 minutes

INGREDIENTS

- 1 large eggplant, sliced into rounds
- 1 can (15 oz) chickpeas, drained and rinsed
- 1 cup cherry tomatoes, halved
- 1/2 cup Kalamata olives, sliced
- 1/4 cup fresh parsley, chopped
- 2 tablespoons olive oil
- 1 tablespoon balsamic vinegar
- 1 teaspoon dried oregano
- Salt and pepper to taste
- Feta cheese crumbles (optional)

DIRECTIONS

1. Preheat the air fryer to 375°F (190°C).
2. In a bowl, toss eggplant slices with olive oil, salt, and pepper.
3. Place the eggplant slices in the air fryer basket in a single layer. Air fry for 8-10 minutes, flipping halfway through, until golden brown and tender.
4. In a separate bowl, combine chickpeas, cherry tomatoes, Kalamata olives, fresh parsley, balsamic vinegar, dried oregano, salt, and pepper.
5. Stack the air-fried eggplant slices with the Mediterranean chickpea mixture.
6. Optionally, sprinkle feta cheese crumbles on top.

Nutritional Information per serving: Calories: 250 | Total Fat: 10g | Saturated Fat: 1g | Trans Fat: 0g | Polyunsaturated Fat: 2g | Monounsaturated Fat: 6g | Cholesterol: 0mg | Sodium: 400mg | Carbohydrates: 35g | Fiber: 12g | Sugars: 8g | Protein: 9g

Garlic Parmesan Zucchini Fries with Marinara Dipping Sauce

🍴 4 servings 🕐 30 minutes

INGREDIENTS

- 3 medium zucchinis, cut into fries
- 1 cup whole wheat breadcrumbs
- 1/2 cup grated Parmesan cheese
- 2 teaspoons garlic powder
- 1 teaspoon dried oregano
- Cooking spray
- 1 cup tomato sauce
- 1 teaspoon olive oil
- 1 clove garlic, minced
- 1/2 teaspoon dried basil
- 1/2 teaspoon dried oregano
- Salt and pepper to taste

DIRECTIONS

1. Preheat the air fryer to 375°F (190°C).
2. In a bowl, combine whole wheat breadcrumbs, grated Parmesan cheese, garlic powder, dried oregano, salt, and pepper.
3. Dip zucchini fries into the breadcrumb mixture, ensuring they are well coated.
4. Place the coated zucchini fries in the air fryer basket in a single layer. Lightly spray with cooking spray.
5. Air fry for 12-15 minutes, shaking the basket halfway through, until the zucchini fries are golden and crispy.
6. In a small saucepan, heat olive oil over medium heat. Add minced garlic and sauté until fragrant.
7. Add tomato sauce, dried basil, dried oregano, salt, and pepper. Simmer for 5-7 minutes.
8. Serve the garlic Parmesan zucchini fries with the marinara dipping sauce.

Nutritional Information per serving: Calories: 180 | Total Fat: 6g | Saturated Fat: 2g | Trans Fat: 0g | Polyunsaturated Fat: 1g | Monounsaturated Fat: 2g | Cholesterol: 6mg | Sodium: 450mg | Carbohydrates: 25g | Fiber: 6g | Sugars: 8g | Protein: 9g

Spicy Paprika and Lime Chicken Skewers

🍴 4 servings 🕐 35 minutes

INGREDIENTS
- 1 pound boneless, skinless chicken breasts, cut into cubes
- 2 tablespoons olive oil
- 1 teaspoon smoked paprika
- 1 teaspoon chili powder
- Zest and juice of 1 lime
- 1 teaspoon cumin
- 1 teaspoon garlic powder
- Salt and pepper to taste
- Wooden skewers, soaked in water for 30 minutes

DIRECTIONS
1. In a bowl, combine olive oil, smoked paprika, chili powder, lime zest, lime juice, cumin, garlic powder, salt, and pepper.
2. Add chicken cubes to the marinade, ensuring they are well-coated. Marinate for at least 15 minutes.
3. Preheat the air fryer to 375°F (190°C).
4.
5. Thread marinated chicken cubes onto the soaked wooden skewers.
6. Place the skewers in the air fryer basket in a single layer.
7. Air fry for 12-15 minutes or until the chicken is cooked through, flipping halfway through.
8. Serve the spicy paprika and lime chicken skewers with your favorite side.

Nutritional Information per serving: Calories: 220 | Total Fat: 11g | Saturated Fat: 2g | Trans Fat: 0g | Polyunsaturated Fat: 2g | Monounsaturated Fat: 6g | Cholesterol: 75mg | Sodium: 90mg | Carbohydrates: 2g | Fiber: 1g | Sugars: 0g | Protein: 26g

Cajun Shrimp and Pineapple Skewers with Avocado Salsa

🍴 4 servings 🕐 30 minutes

INGREDIENTS
- 1 pound large shrimp, peeled and deveined
- 1 tablespoon olive oil
- 1 tablespoon Cajun seasoning
- 1 teaspoon garlic powder
- 1 teaspoon paprika
- 1/2 teaspoon onion powder
- Wooden skewers, soaked in water for 30 minutes
- 2 ripe avocados, diced
- 1 cup pineapple, diced
- 1/4 cup red onion, finely chopped
- 1/4 cup fresh cilantro, chopped
- Juice of 1 lime
- Salt and pepper to taste

DIRECTIONS
1. In a bowl, combine olive oil, Cajun seasoning, garlic powder, paprika, onion powder, salt, and pepper.
2. Add shrimp to the marinade, ensuring they are well-coated. Marinate for at least 15 minutes.
3. Preheat the air fryer to 375°F (190°C).
4. Thread marinated shrimp onto the soaked wooden skewers.
5. Place the skewers in the air fryer basket in a single layer.
6. Air fry for 8-10 minutes or until the shrimp are opaque and cooked through, flipping halfway through.
7. In a bowl, combine diced avocados, diced pineapple, chopped red onion, cilantro, lime juice, salt, and pepper.
8. Serve Cajun shrimp skewers over rice or with the avocado salsa on the side.

Nutritional Information per serving: Calories: 280 | Total Fat: 16g | Saturated Fat: 2g | Trans Fat: 0g | Polyunsaturated Fat: 2g | Monounsaturated Fat: 10g | Cholesterol: 160mg | Sodium: 220mg | Carbohydrates: 16g | Fiber: 7g | Sugars: 6g | Protein: 22g

Sesame Ginger Tofu Nuggets with Sriracha Mayo

🍴 4 servings 🕐 40 minutes

INGREDIENTS
- 1 block extra-firm tofu, pressed and cut into nuggets
- 2 tablespoons soy sauce
- 1 tablespoon rice vinegar
- 1 tablespoon sesame oil
- 1 tablespoon grated ginger
- 1 tablespoon cornstarch
- 2 tablespoons sesame seeds
- Cooking spray
- 1/2 cup light mayonnaise
- 2 tablespoons Sriracha sauce
- 1 tablespoon lime juice

DIRECTIONS

1. In a bowl, whisk together soy sauce, rice vinegar, sesame oil, grated ginger, and cornstarch.
2. Dip tofu nuggets into the marinade, ensuring they are well-coated. Marinate for at least 15 minutes.
3. Preheat the air fryer to 375°F (190°C).
4. In a separate bowl, coat marinated tofu nuggets with sesame seeds.
5. Place the tofu nuggets in the air fryer basket in a single layer. Lightly spray with cooking spray.
6. Air fry for 12-15 minutes or until the tofu is golden and crispy, flipping halfway through.
7. In a small bowl, mix together light mayonnaise, Sriracha sauce, and lime juice.
8. Serve sesame ginger tofu nuggets with Sriracha mayo for dipping.

Nutritional Information per serving: Calories: 220 | Total Fat: 14g | Saturated Fat: 2g | Trans Fat: 0g | Polyunsaturated Fat: 6g | Monounsaturated Fat: 5g | Cholesterol: 0mg | Sodium: 450mg | Carbohydrates: 13g | Fiber: 3g | Sugars: 2g | Protein: 14g

CONCLUSION

In the journey towards optimal heart health, the "Heart Healthy Cookbook for Beginners" serves as your trusted companion. This cookbook is more than a collection of recipes; it's a transformative guide designed to make heart-healthy living both accessible and delightful.

As we conclude this culinary exploration, it's evident that nourishing our hearts involves more than just ingredients – it's a lifestyle. The importance of a heart-healthy diet cannot be overstated, and this cookbook is crafted to empower you with the knowledge and flavors needed to embark on this transformative journey.

Understanding heart health, from managing cholesterol to maintaining optimal blood pressure, becomes a breeze with the insights shared in these pages. The key components of heart-healthy foods, coupled with tips on how to read nutritional labels, ensure that you make informed choices for your cardiovascular well-being.

The heart of this cookbook lies not only in its delectable recipes but also in its commitment to making heart-healthy cooking and meal planning an enjoyable part of your routine. With practical tips and a 4-week meal plan, the cookbook simplifies the path to a heart-healthy lifestyle, helping you cultivate habits that last a lifetime.

Here's to heart-healthy living and savoring the delicious possibilities of a nourished heart!

4-WEEK MEAL PLAN

Meal planner

for a week 1

	BREAKFAST	LUNCH	DINNER	SNACKS
MON	Oatmeal with Blueberries and Chia Seeds	Grilled Chicken and Quinoa Salad	Garlic Lemon Herb Chicken	Baked Sweet Potato Fries with Avocado Dip
TUE	Avocado Toast on Whole Grain Bread	Lentil and Vegetable Soup	Grilled Trout with Herb Salad	Pear and Ricotta Cheese on Multigrain Crackers
WED	Greek Yogurt Parfait with Mixed Berries and Almonds	Avocado and Turkey Lettuce Wraps	Baked Eggplant with Tomato and Feta	Hummus with Sliced Cucumber and Carrots
THU	Quinoa Breakfast Bowl with Nuts and Apples	Mediterranean Chickpea Salad	Roasted Red Pepper and Lentil Soup	Fresh Fruit Salad with Mint and Lime
FRI	Spinach and Mushroom Egg White Omelet	Baked Salmon with Steamed Broccoli	Stuffed Acorn Squash with Quinoa and Kale	Crispy Baked Zucchini Chips
SAT	Banana Walnut Overnight Oats	Whole Wheat Pasta Primavera	Rosemary Lemon Baked Cod	Sunflower Seed and Cranberry Energy Bites
SUN	Smoked Salmon and Avocado Whole Wheat Bagel	Tuna Salad Stuffed Tomatoes	Mushroom and Barley Soup	Whole Grain Rice Cakes with Almond Butter and Berries

Meal planner
for a week 2

	BREAKFAST	LUNCH	DINNER	SNACKS
MON	Almond Butter and Banana Smoothie	Veggie Hummus Wrap	Lemon Pepper Cod with Zucchini Noodles	Spinach and Feta Stuffed Mushrooms
TUE	Kale and Red Pepper Mini Frittatas	Roasted Red Pepper and Spinach Panini	Turkey and Spinach Meatballs in Marinara Sauce	Cucumber Boats Filled with Tuna Salad
WED	Steel-Cut Oats with Pomegranate Seeds	Butternut Squash and Kale Stir-Fry	Baked Tilapia with Mango Salsa	Baked Sweet Potato Fries with Avocado Dip
THU	Chia Seed Pudding with Kiwi and Coconut	Black Bean and Corn Salad	Sesame Ginger Stir-Fry with Tofu	Pear and Ricotta Cheese on Multigrain Crackers
FRI	Whole Grain Pancakes with Fresh Fruit Compote	Grilled Vegetable and Goat Cheese Sandwich	Kale and White Bean Soup	Hummus with Sliced Cucumber and Carrots
SAT	Cottage Cheese with Pineapple and Flaxseeds	Cauliflower Rice Burrito Bowl	Lemon Herb Roasted Chicken and Potatoes	Fresh Fruit Salad with Mint and Lime
SUN	Baked Sweet Potato Hash with Peppers and Onions	Shrimp and Avocado Salad	Vegetarian Stuffed Zucchini Boats	Crispy Baked Zucchini Chips

Meal planner
for a week 3

	BREAKFAST	LUNCH	DINNER	SNACKS
MON	Raspberry Almond Muffins (made with oat flour)	Halibut with Tomato Basil Salsa	Grilled Lemon-Herb Chicken Skewers	Sunflower Seed and Cranberry Energy Bites
TUE	Turkey and Spinach Breakfast Burritos (using whole wheat tortillas)	Turkey and Spinach Meatballs in Marinara Sauce	Stuffed Chicken Breast with Spinach and Ricotta	Whole Grain Rice Cakes with Almond Butter and Berries
WED	Poached Eggs over Sautéed Greens and Whole Grain Toast	Rosemary Garlic Roasted Chicken	Slow-Cooked Beef and Vegetable Stew	Baked Sweet Potato Fries with Avocado Dip
THU	Berry and Spinach Smoothie with Soy Milk	Honey Mustard Glazed Chicken Thighs	Grilled Turkey Burgers with Avocado	Pear and Ricotta Cheese on Multigrain Crackers
FRI	Pear and Walnut Baked Oatmeal	Balsamic Honey Skillet Chicken	Asian-Style Turkey Lettuce Wraps	Hummus with Sliced Cucumber and Carrots
SAT	Savory Quinoa and Vegetable Breakfast Bowls	Spiced Chicken and Sweet Potato Bowl	Pork Tenderloin with Herbed Quinoa	Fresh Fruit Salad with Mint and Lime
SUN	Whole Grain Waffles with Sliced Peaches and Honey	Moroccan Spiced Lamb Chops	Chicken and Black Bean Burrito Bow	Crispy Baked Zucchini Chips

Meal planner
for a week 4

	BREAKFAST	LUNCH	DINNER	SNACKS
MON	Mediterranean Scramble with Tomatoes, Olives, and Feta	Grilled Salmon with Mango Salsa	Lemon Pepper Cod with Zucchini Noodles	Spinach and Feta Stuffed Mushrooms
TUE	Multigrain Porridge with Dates and Spices	Shrimp and Asparagus Stir Fry	Baked Haddock with Herbed Crumbs	Cucumber Boats Filled with Tuna Salad
WED	Apple Cinnamon Breakfast Barley	Spicy Tuna and Avocado Cucumber Sushi Rolls	Seared Scallops with Quinoa and Spinach	Baked Sweet Potato Fries with Avocado Dip
THU	Zucchini and Carrot Breakfast Muffins	Mediterranean Shrimp and Orzo Salad	Teriyaki Glazed Salmon Bowl	Pear and Ricotta Cheese on Multigrain Crackers
FRI	Warm Millet Cereal with Cinnamon Apples	Blackened Tilapia with Cilantro Lime Slaw	Seafood Paella with Brown Rice	Hummus with Sliced Cucumber and Carrots
SAT	Tomato and Basil Breakfast Bruschetta	Crab and Avocado Salad	Pan-Seared Trout with Almond Butter	Fresh Fruit Salad with Mint and Lime
SUN	Peanut Butter and Strawberry Chia Jam on Sprouted Grain Bread	Miso Soup with Salmon and Bok Choy	Garlic Lemon Shrimp Skewers	Crispy Baked Zucchini Chips

Shopping list
for a week 3

✔	Product	Quantity	✔	Product	Quantity
☐	Raspberries	1 cup	☐	Halibut fillets	2-3
☐	Oat flour	1 lb	☐	Fresh basil	1 bunch
☐	Tomatoes	3-4	☐	Chicken breasts (for skewers)	3-4
☐	Lemons	2-3	☐	Ground turkey	2 lbs
☐	Whole wheat tortillas	1 pack	☐	Marinara sauce	1 jar
☐	Spinach	2 large bags	☐	Whole grain rice cakes	1 pack
☐	Ricotta cheese	1 cup	☐	Mixed berries	1-2 cups
☐	Almond butter	1 jar	☐	Mixed greens	1 bag
☐	Eggs	1 dozen	☐	Rosemary	1 bunch
☐	Whole grain bread	1 loaf	☐	Beef (for stew)	1 lb
☐	Garlic	1 bulb	☐	Sweet potatoes	2-3 medium
☐	Mixed vegetables (for stew)	2-3 cups	☐	Honey	As needed
☐	Soy milk	1 quart	☐	Chicken thighs	4-6 pieces
☐	Mustard	1 bottle	☐	Avocado	2-3
☐	Turkey burgers	1 pack	☐	Walnuts	1/2 cup
☐	Pears	2-3	☐	Balsamic vinegar	1 bottle
☐	Oats (rolled)	1-2 cups	☐	Chicken (for bowl)	1 lb
☐	Quinoa	1 cup	☐	Fresh fruit (assorted for salad)	2-3 cups
☐	Pork tenderloin	1-2 lbs	☐	Whole grain waffles	1 box
☐	Mint	1 small bunch	☐	Lamb chops	4-6 pieces
☐	Peaches	2-3	☐	Black beans (canned or dry)	1 can or 1/2 lb
☐	Moroccan spices	1 small jar	☐	Multigrain crackers	1 box
☐	Zucchini	2 medium	☐	Salt, pepper, garlic powder, etc.	As needed
☐	Hummus	1 container	☐		
☐	Carrots	2-3	☐		
☐	Cucumber	2-3	☐		
☐	Olive oil	As needed	☐		
☐	Almonds	1/2 cup	☐		

Shopping list
for a week 4

✔	Product	Quantity
☐	Eggs	1 dozen
☐	Black olives	1 jar
☐	Salmon fillets	2-3
☐	Cod fillets	2-3
☐	Zucchini	3-4
☐	Dates	1 cup
☐	Shrimp	1 lb
☐	Haddock fillets	2-3
☐	Apples	2-3
☐	Tuna (canned)	2 cans
☐	Sushi nori sheets	1 pack
☐	Quinoa	1 cup
☐	Carrots	2-3
☐	Orzo pasta	1 lb
☐	Pears	2-3
☐	Multigrain crackers	1 box
☐	Tilapia fillets	2-3
☐	Limes	2 3
☐	Seafood mix (for paella)	1 lb
☐	Fresh basil	1 bunch
☐	Trout fillets	2-3
☐	Fresh fruit (assorted for salad)	2-3 cups
☐	Sprouted grain bread	1 loaf
☐	Strawberry jam	1 jar
☐	Miso paste	1 jar
☐	Salt, pepper, garlic powder, etc.	As needed
☐	Garlic	1 bulb
☐	Cucumber	2-3

✔	Product	Quantity
☐	Zucchini (for chips)	2 medium
☐	Tomatoes	3-4
☐	Feta cheese	1 cup
☐	Mango	1
☐	Lemon pepper seasoning	As needed
☐	Multigrain cereal or oats	1 box
☐	Spices (cinnamon, nutmeg, etc.)	As needed
☐	Asparagus	1 bunch
☐	Panko breadcrumbs	1 cup
☐	Barley	1 cup
☐	Avocado	2-3
☐	Scallops	1 lb
☐	Sweet potatoes	2-3 medium
☐	Whole grain flour	1 lb
☐	Teriyaki sauce	1 bottle
☐	Ricotta cheese	1 cup
☐	Millet	1 cup
☐	Cilantro	1 bunch
☐	Brown rice	1 lb
☐	Tomatoes (for bruschetta)	2-3
☐	Crab meat	1/2 lb
☐	Almond butter	1 jar
☐	Peanut butter	1 jar
☐	Chia seeds	1/4 cup
☐	Mint	1 small bunch
☐	Bok choy	1-2 heads
☐	Hummus	1 container
☐	Olive oil	As needed

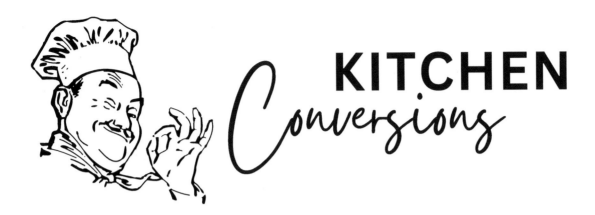

KITCHEN
Conversions

VOLUME CONVERSIONS

- 1 tablespoon (tbsp) = 3 teaspoons (tsp)
- 1 fluid ounce (fl oz) = 2 tablespoons (tbsp)
- 1 cup = 8 fluid ounces
- 1 pint (pt) = 2 cups
- 1 quart (qt) = 2 pints
- 1 gallon (gal) = 4 quarts

  - 1 cup = 240 milliliters (ml)
  - 1 tablespoon (tbsp) = 15 milliliters
  - 1 teaspoon (tsp) = 5 milliliters
  - 1 fluid ounce (fl oz) = 29 milliliters
  - 1 pint (pt) = 473 milliliters
  - 1 quart (qt) = 946 milliliters
  - 1 gallon (gal) = 4 milliliters

WEIGHT CONVERSIONS

- 1 ounce (oz) = 28 grams (g)
- 1 pound (lb) = 16 ounces
- 1 kilogram (kg) = 2.2 pounds

OVEN TEMPERATURE CONVERSIONS

- Moderate oven: $350°F = 180°C$
- Moderate to Hot oven: $375°F = 190°C$
- Hot oven: $400°F = 200°C$
- Very Hot oven: $425°F = 220°C$

COMMON INGREDIENT EQUIVALENTS

- 1 stick of butter = 1/2 cup = 8 tablespoons
- 1 cup of flour = 120 grams
- 1 cup of sugar = 200 grams
- 1 cup of brown sugar (packed) = 220 grams

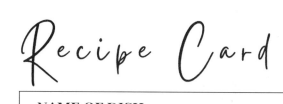

Recipe Card

NAME OF DISH :		
SERVES :	PREP TIME :	COOK TIME :

INGREDIENTS

_____

_____

_____

_____

_____

_____

_____

INGREDIENTS

_____

_____

_____

_____

_____

_____

_____

DIRECTIONS

_____

_____

_____

_____

_____

_____

_____

_____

_____

_____

_____

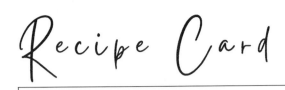

NAME OF DISH :		
SERVES :	PREP TIME :	COOK TIME :

INGREDIENTS

_____

_____

_____

_____

_____

_____

_____

_____

INGREDIENTS

_____

_____

_____

_____

_____

_____

_____

_____

DIRECTIONS

_____

_____

_____

_____

_____

_____

_____

_____

_____

_____

_____

_____

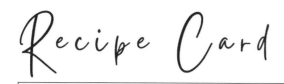

NAME OF DISH :		
SERVES :	PREP TIME :	COOK TIME :

INGREDIENTS

_____

_____

_____

_____

_____

_____

_____

_____

INGREDIENTS

_____

_____

_____

_____

_____

_____

_____

_____

DIRECTIONS

_____

_____

_____

_____

_____

_____

_____

_____

_____

_____

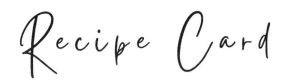

NAME OF DISH :		
SERVES :	PREP TIME :	COOK TIME :

INGREDIENTS

_____

_____

_____

_____

_____

_____

_____

INGREDIENTS

_____

_____

_____

_____

_____

_____

_____

DIRECTIONS

_____

_____

_____

_____

_____

_____

_____

_____

_____

_____

_____

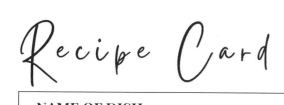

NAME OF DISH :		
SERVES :	PREP TIME :	COOK TIME :

INGREDIENTS

_____

_____

_____

_____

_____

_____

_____

_____

INGREDIENTS

_____

_____

_____

_____

_____

_____

_____

_____

DIRECTIONS

_____

_____

_____

_____

_____

_____

_____

_____

_____

_____

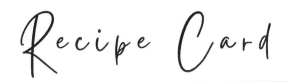

Recipe Card

NAME OF DISH :		
SERVES :	PREP TIME :	COOK TIME :

INGREDIENTS

_____

_____

_____

_____

_____

_____

_____

INGREDIENTS

_____

_____

_____

_____

_____

_____

_____

DIRECTIONS

_____

_____

_____

_____

_____

_____

_____

_____

_____

_____

_____

BLOOD PRESSURE MONITORING LIST

Date	Systolic	Diastolic	Meds taken	Well being / Notes

Date	Systolic	Diastolic	Meds taken	Well being / Notes

Date	Systolic	Diastolic	Meds taken	Well being / Notes

Made in the USA
Columbia, SC
21 April 2024

34671454R00057